50 OSCEs In Su

Candidate Briefings, Actor I

Louise Merker MBChB MRCS

Pippa Leighton MBBS MRCS

Jamie Crichton MBChB MRCS

© 2016 MD+ Publishing

Published by: MD+ Publishing

Cover Design: Alexander Logan

ISBN-10: 0993113893

ISBN-13: 978-0993113895

Printed in the United Kingdom

CONTENTS

Preface

Chapter 1: Communication

Chapter 2: OSCEs

Chapter 3: Vivas

MORE ONLINE

www.mrcspartbquestions.com

 Access Over 1000 More MRCS Questions

Head over to the MRCS Part B website for our online MRCS Part B questions bank featuring over 1000 unique, interactive MRCS scenarios with comprehensive answers.

Created by high scoring, successful trainees the website and question bank can be accessed from your home computer, laptop or mobile device making your preparation as easy and convenient as possible.

About This Workbook

This book was written by three surgical trainees with the intention of creating realistic scenarios to revise for the Intercollegiate MRCS Part B OSCE. We wrote it a few years after sitting the exam, having been through the process and feeling that we needed a modern reading resource for practice with colleagues or alone. With the help of speciality surgeons and experts, we put together a series of stations that reflect the nature of the reformed exam, and provide a basis for realistic revision at home. The book is simple and easy to use.

The book is split into three parts:

1.Communication
Clinical histories and communication skills

2. OSCE
Clinical examinations and procedural skills

3. Viva
Direct examiner questions on applied science, surgical pathology and critical care

The book works best when used in pairs or groups; with one candidate, an examiner and another acting as the patient if required.

Each station closely follows the exam structure. There is an initial vignette, mimicking the instructions you will receive in the exam. Then follows a simulated patient description for those stations requiring an actor. Finally there is an examiner marking sheet, with a defined algorithm that closely matches the formal exam mark sheet including additional supplementary questions.

The stations should be run with similar timings to the actual exam. The candidate vignettes should be read within 1 minute. An OSCE or communication station should be completed within 6 minutes, with 3 minutes for findings presentation and questions, and a viva station should be completed within 9 minutes. This will give an accurate representation of the timings on exam day.
The book is not comprehensive because the aim is to focus mainly on exam technique. There are relatively fewer stations on clinical pathology and anatomy. There are some fantastic books and online resources that cover these topics at the level required for the exam. We have listed these at the end of this chapter.

About The MRCS Part B OSCE

The modern MRCS Part B exam is described below. There is a very useful 'Guide to the MRCS examination' document freely available on the websites for the surgical colleges. It contains a comprehensive syllabus, recommended reading textbooks and a description of the Part B structure and assessment matrix. It also contains a range of example questions and their mark sheets. We recommend you read this document in detail. It is important to highlight the exam is essentially the same regardless of what college you are taking it with.

A. PREPARATION
This examination requires 4 – 6 months of dedicated revision. This is a long exam, around 4 hours of constant concentration, so it is very important to maintain good physical and mental health in the run up.

B. STRUCTURE
The Part B exam tests clinical acumen and applied scientific knowledge, to assess the ability to integrate and apply knowledge. The stations reflect daily surgical activity, and the emphasis is on a demonstration of basic safe practice and competence. There are 18 stations each 10 minutues long in total with 2 rest stations in each half of the exam. Each station has an examiner, with some stations requiring two to assess separate skills e.g. communication and technical skill.

Stations are in the following categories:

Anatomy and surgical pathology (5 stations)
Applied science and critical care (3 stations)
Communication skills (4 stations)
Clinical and procedural skills (6 stations)

C. MARKS
Assessment is based on four main domains, which reflect the GMC's 'Good Medical Practice':
*   Clinical knowledge and application
*   Clinical and technical skill
*   Communication
*   Professionalism

There are 20 marks available per station. Stations are weighted towards particular domains, with the overall exam reflecting an equal weight in each domain. Each station has a structured mark sheet to guide examiners. There is also an overall judgement mark that each examiner gives on the student performance (Pass, Borderline, Fail), reflecting an overall impression of the student.

Of note, we found that the structure of the exam gave very little time for elaboration, and so the marks were very clearly given to concise answers containing only relevant phrases.

D. BASICS
Dress smart: suits and white shirts
Remember, the examiners have seen many candidates over the years. They are looking for safe surgeons; they do not like the flashy trainee who wants to show off. Be safe and sensible, and you will pass.

BOOKS WE USED
Below is a list of the most useful books we read during our revision:

Advanced Trauma Life Support (ATLS) Student Course Manual. American College of Surgeons 2012.
Fishman J, Elwell VA, Chowdhury R. OSCEs for the MRCS Part B A Bailey & Love Revision Guide: A Bailey and Love Revision Guide. CRC Press 2009.
Kanani M. Surgical Critical Care Vivas. Cambridge University Press 2002.
O. James Garden, Andrew W. Bradbury, John L. R. Forsythe and Rowan W. Parks. Principles and Practice of Surgery. 5th Edition. Chuchill Livingstone Elsevier 2007.

We hope you find this book as useful as we did creating it.

Good luck,

Louise, Pippa and Jamie

Glossary

ABG	Arterial blood gas
ARDS	Acute respiratory distress syndrome
ASGBI	Association of Surgeons of Great Britain and Ireland
COPD	Chronic obstructive pulmonary disease
CTPA	CT pulmonary angiography
CXR	Chest x-ray
DH	Drug history
ECG	Electrocardiogram
ED	Emergency department
ERCP	Endoscopic retrograde cholangio-pancreatography
FBC	Full blood count
FH	Family history
ICE	Ideas, concerns, expectations
IVI	Intravenous infusion
LRTI	Lower respiratory tract infection
MI	Myocardial infarction
NSAIDs	Non-steroidal anti-inflammatory drugs
PE	Pulmonary embolus
PMH	Past medical history
SH	Social history
STEMI	ST-segment elevation myocardial infarction
U&E	Urea and electrolytes
UO	Urine output

1 COMMUNICATION

COMMUNICATION

1.1 | Back Pain History

 Candidate Briefing

Mr/Mrs Jones is a 45 year-old who has presents to A&E complaining of acute lower back pain. Please take a history from him/her, present your findings to the examiner and answer their questions.

 Actor Briefing

You are Mr/Mrs Jones. You had sudden onset lower back pain when getting out of your car. It came on about 3 hours ago.
The pain is in the centre of your back and it travels down the back of both legs, the right more than the left. It is worse if you move, cough or sneeze.

You are able to walk but it is painful.

You have not had any urinary or faecal incontinence but it felt a bit strange when you went for a pee earlier. If pressed on this by the candidate, explain you're not really sure what it was, but you didn't really feel like you needed to go, but you urinated a large volume and you had to check to see that you had finished as you weren't really aware of it.

You are not sure if it feels numb around your perineum.
You have had niggly back pain going into your buttock on and off for many years but never this bad.
You have no pain higher up your spine
You have not lost any weight recently, though you are a bit overweight.
You have no pain in your abdomen/chest. You feel well in yourself.

PMH: Nil

DH: allergic to penicillin. Nil regular

SH: Smokes 10 cigarettes a day. Drinks 3-4 glasses of wine on a Friday night. Independent shop assistant. Lives with husband and two cats

Systems Review: Nil of note

ICE: You are in a lot of discomfort and want something doing about it.

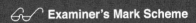
Examiner's Mark Scheme

History Taking	Mark (0-4)			
Introduction • Introduces self to patient, confirms patient identity, explains role and establishes a rapport				
Presenting Complaint • Elicits necessary information from patient • Uses appropriate open questions • Takes a comprehensive history from a patient				
Red Flag Symptoms • Accurately identifies and interprets key clinical features • Specific red flag symptoms to cover are leg weakness/neurology, bowel/bladder symptoms, weight loss, thoracic pain and night pain				
PMH, DH, SH and systems review • Has a systematic approach and covers key information				

Presenting The History	Mark (0-4)			
Summarises • Accurately summarises a well-structured history. • Accurately describes key clinical symptoms. • Interprets key clinical signs. • Appreciates the potential seriousness of the history- could this be cauda equina?				

Clinical Knowledge	Mark (0-4)			
Formulates A Diagnosis and Plan • Able to give a differential diagnosis based on the history. • Differentials would be prolapsed disc, exacerbation of osteoarthritis, spinal stenosis, spinal fracture or most importantly cauda equina • Appropriate investigations would include MRI spine (urgent if cauda equina suspected)				

COMMUNICATION

COMMUNICATION

Communication Skills	Mark (0-4)			
Introduction • Uses appropriate opening/introductions and establishes purpose of the interview.				
Language • Uses technical/non-technical language appropriately, accurately and with fluency. • Adapts language/behaviour as needed and adjusts style of questioning (open/closed) as appropriate, with good rapport and appropriate body language. • Clear communication.				
Listening and Rapport • Establishes relationship of respect with patient. • Demonstrates active listening.				
Empathy • Demonstrates empathy and responds appropriately to patient's concerns and questions.				
Closure and Timing • Adequate closure of interview. • Closes within allocated time.				

Professionalism	Mark (0-4)			
Overall Conduct • Plans ahead, identifying requirements and prioritising accordingly. • Good time management. • Appreciates need for further investigation • Is sympathetic to this patient's problems.				

Follow On Questions

What are your differential diagnoses?
Need to be suspicious for acute cauda equina. Other possibilities include disc prolapse, fracture, bone tumour or muscular strain/spasm

How do you wish to proceed?
Thorough examination including neurology, anal tone and peri-anal sensation
Imaging: patient likely needs an urgent MRI spine

At what vertebral level does the spinal cord terminate? How can this be identified using surface anatomy?
It terminates around the level of L1/2. The L1 vertebral body is in the trans-pyloric plane, which is halfway between the suprasternal notch and the pubic symphysis

Examiner's Overall Assessment		
Pass	Fail	Borderline

TOP TIPS

✚ Cauda equina syndrome is an emergency and failure to identify and decompress CES within 48hrs of onset can lead to chronic bowel, bladder and motor dysfunction

✚ When asking about urinary symptoms find out whether the patient can feel if their bladder is full, can feel themselves urination and can start and stop the stream. If not this implies sacral nerve involvement.

✚ Bilateral leg neurology, urinary symptoms and a progression of symptoms acutely requires an urgent MRI.

✚ Don't forget the red flags of back pain: fever, weight loss, constant pain, night pain, bowel and bladder dysfunction, new back pain at the extremes of age and history of malignancy.

1.2 | Breaking Bad News

 Candidate Briefing

You are the night SHO on-call for surgery. Overnight you assessed a patient who had undergone an angioplasty earlier that day for claudication of his right calf. Unfortunately when you assessed him he had a large haematoma and was haemodynamically comprised. He has been taken back to theatre by the vascular consultant and your registrar to treat a possible retroperitoneal haematoma. You have been called to talk to the patient's wife who has just come in to visit him.

 Actor Briefing

You are Mrs B the elderly wife of Mr B. You have come in to visit him this morning early before going to the shops and he isn't in his bed space.

You are very anxious and concerned and do not understand why he is "back in theatre" as the nurse has told you as he only came in for a little procedure under local anaesthetic to ease his leg pain.

You have a daughter locally but she is currently on holiday in Spain. You do not fully grasp the severity of the situation.

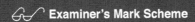 **Examiner's Mark Scheme**

Introduction	Mark (0-4)			
Opening • Candidate should introduce themselves to the patient including their name and role • They should check the visitors name and their relationship to the patient				
Confidentiality • Some acknowledgement of patient confidentiality should be made. Ideally they should say something along the line of "I would normally check if the patient was happy for me to discuss their medical treatment with you but given the situation this isn't possible" • This is acknowledging that patient's have full confidentiality to their treatment even from close family if they wish.				

Breaking Bad News	Mark (0-4)			
Checks Understanding • The candidate should first check what the relative's understanding of the situation is.				
Addresses Concerns •They should address any immediate concerns of the relative e.g. is my husband alive?				
Explanation • The candidate should provide a satisfactory explanation of the events overnight and what is happening to the patient currently e.g he has had to be taken back to theatre to stop the bleeding				

COMMUNICATION

COMMUNICATION

Communication Skills	Mark (0-4)			
Introduction • Uses appropriate opening/introductions and establishes purpose of the interview. • Confirms that there is common understanding				
Language • Uses technical/non-technical language appropriately, accurately and with fluency. • Adapts language/behaviour as needed and adjusts style of questioning (open/closed) as appropriate, with good rapport and appropriate body language. • Clear communication. • Uses warning shot to hint that the news is not good before delivering the news directly				
Listening and Rapport • Establishes relationship of respect with patient. • Demonstrates active listening. • Allows silence and time for relative to process information				
Empathy • The candidate should be sympathetic toward the patient and repeat information as needed being aware the patient may not understand medical jargon. • The candidate should offer the relative further support in terms of contacting friends or family to support them.				
Closure and Timing • Adequate closure of interview. • Closes within allocated time.				

Professionalism	Mark (0-4)			
Overall Conduct • Able to recognise and manage complex and competing needs. • Good time management. • Is empathetic to the relative's needs				

Follow On Questions

Ideally how should bad news be broken?

Quiet room away from the main ward with seating, bleep or telephones switched off, take a nurse for support for both yourself and the patient, have tissues or water handy. Senior support if available or at least discussed the case with the consultant or senior registrar.

The relative is annoyed they weren't called overnight. How would you respond to this?

Firstly apologise. Then suggest it may have been forgotten due to the emergency of the situation. State that you will raise the issue with the night team and put a note that relatives want to be contacted at all hours. Offer them PALs information.

What should you do immediately after this discussion with the relative?

Document the meeting in the patient's notes or on a history sheet if the notes are in theatre.

Examiner's Overall Assessment		
Pass	Fail	Borderline

TOP TIPS

➕ Use a 'warning shot' to prepare the relative before delivering the bad news. This might be a lead-in sentence such as 'Unfortunately it is not good news, I am sorry to tell you that...'

➕ Be prepared for the actor to go silent or cry following receiving the news. Do not be afraid to allow for silence, rather give the actor time to process the news before offering support.

➕ Involving MDT members and 'safety-netting' by arranging a further conversation with the relatives is a nice way to close the scenario.

COMMUNICATION

1.3 | Breast Pain

 Candidate Briefing

Mrs Beeton is a 30 year-old lady who has been referred to the two-week wait breast clinic by her GP with a history of breast pain. Please take her history then answer the examiner's questions

 Actor Briefing

You are Ms Beal. You should come across as very anxious.

You went to see your GP last week because you have been getting pain in your breasts on and off for the last 2 months. It is worse in the right than the left; it feels like a nagging ache all the time. If asked specifically, it is worse around the time of your periods. You have not noticed any lumps but you do not self-examine. You have had no changes in the size or shape of your breasts, no skin changes and no nipple discharge nor retraction.

You feel well in yourself but extremely anxious as your mother had breast cancer and had to have a mastectomy aged 67. You have not lost any weight or had any pain elsewhere. Your menstrual cycle is regular. You have no children and you have a regular partner.

PMH: Nil. Specifically no history of breast/gynaecological malignancy

DH: Allergic to penicillin. You take the oral contraceptive pill – on specific questioning, it is the combined pill

SH: You smoke 5-6 cigarettes a day and drink 3-4 glasses of cider a week. You are fit and active, working as a personal trainer at a gym.

FH: Mother breast cancer. No other history of breast or ovarian cancer

Systems review: Nil

ICE: Very anxious that this is cancer. You are very keen for a mammogram to rule it out.

COMMUNICATION

Examiner's Mark Scheme

History Taking	Mark (0-4)			
Introduction • Introduces self to patient and explains role				
Presenting Complaint • Elicits necessary information from patient • Accurately identifies and interprets key clinical features • Elicits breast pain in both breasts for 2 months intermittently, cyclical with no lumps.				
Breast Pain History • Asks relevant questions for a breast assessment such as any lumps felt, nipple changes, skin changes, OCP or HRT use, smoking status, previous mammograms				
PMH, DH, SH and systems review • Elicits positive family history • Picks up on patient's anxiety • Has a systematic approach. • Addresses patient's, ideas, concerns and expectations				

Clinical Knowledge/Presenting	Mark (0-4)			
Presenting the History • Presents a well-structured history. • Key features are breast pain being cyclical or non-cyclical, any lumps present, any skin changes or nipple tethering, history of nipple discharge • Accurately describes key clinical symptoms.				
Clinical Knowledge • Understands key clinical signs. • Able to use history to suggest a sensible management plan such as clinical examination and US. • Mammogram is inappropriate as the patient is less than 40 years old • Suggests a differential diagnosis of mastalgia, musculoskeletal chest pain or underlying malignancy				

COMMUNICATION

Communication Skills	Mark (0-4)			
Introduction • Uses appropriate opening/introductions and establishes purpose of the interview. • Ascertains what the patient already knows				
Language • Uses technical/non-technical language appropriately, accurately and with fluency. • Adapts language/behaviour as needed and adjusts style of questioning (open/closed) as appropriate, with good rapport and appropriate body language. • Clear communication.				
Listening and Rapport • Establishes relationship of respect with patient. • Demonstrates active listening. • Does not worry patient excessively with possible diagnosis at this stage – need to await results of investigations.				
Empathy • Demonstrates empathy and responds appropriately to patient's concerns and questions. • Aware of patient's anxiety				
Closure and Timing • Adequate closure of interview. • Closes within allocated time.				

Professionalism	Mark (0-4)			
Overall Conduct • Good time and resource management. • Appreciates need for further investigation • Is sympathetic to this patient's problems.				

Follow On Questions

What are you differential diagnoses?

The important thing to exclude here is breast cancer. Benign breast pain is extremely common and probably the most likely cause, but is a diagnosis of exclusion. Its aetiology is not well-understood but it may be related to hormone changes during the menstrual cycle. Musculoskeletal pain is a possibility given her occupation. Other things to think about include mastitis if she were breast-feeding, abscesses (unlikely if bilateral) and fibrocystic disease.

At what ages are women invited to the breast cancer screening program in the UK?

Currently the screening program invites women aged 50 to 70 to the program, though this is being extended to 47 to 73.

How will you investigate her here in clinic?

The default is triple assessment – examination, imaging and, if appropriate, tissue biopsy. Because she is young her breast tissue will be dense and so a mammogram is less useful – ultrasound is a better choice.

Examiner's Overall Assessment		
Pass	Fail	Borderline

COMMUNICATION

TOP TIPS

 This woman is extremely anxious, reassurance and a calm approach are key.

 Make sure you take a full breast assessment history with any breast symptoms.

1.4 | Cancelled Operation

 Candidate Briefing

You are the surgical SHO on-call. Mr/Mrs X is a 22 year-old patient with a clinical diagnosis of appendicitis. He/she has been booked, consented and is awaiting a laparoscopic appendicectomy. It is now 5pm. You have just been to A&E where you saw a 65 year-old presenting with a ruptured abdominal aortic aneurysm (AAA). The vascular consultant is aware and is being rushed to the only available emergency theatre. The laparoscopic appendicectomy will need to be postponed until tomorrow as there is no chance it will be done tonight. Go to the ward to explain this to Mr/Mrs X.

 Actor Briefing

You are Mr/Mrs X, a 22 year old who presented 2 days ago with a gradual onset central abdominal pain that now localises to the right lower abdomen.

You understand that the doctors were keeping an eye on you to see how things went, but since they have got worse they have decided you have appendicitis and want to do an operation.

You were expecting to have your operation today and have been fasting since midnight. It is now 5pm and so you are very keen to get it over with.

You should act understandably frustrated when the candidate explains the operation has been cancelled. If they deliver the news particularly badly, give them a bit of a hard time.

Questions you may ask:
• Why am I not being done urgently? Why does this other case take priority?
• What are the risks of postponing the surgery till tomorrow?
• What happens if I get worse?
• Is there no chance of me being done after this emergency case?
• Can you promise me I will be done tomorrow?
• Can I eat now?
• If there is no rush to do the operation, can I not go home and come back for it in the next few days/weeks?

COMMUNICATION

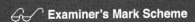 Examiner's Mark Scheme

Introduction	Mark (0-4)			
Opening • Introduces self to patient including name and role • Establishes that they are speaking to the correct patient				

Cancelling The Patient	Mark (0-4)			
Gathers Information • Finds out what the patient knows so far • "What do you think the current situation is?"				
Explanation of Cancellation • Clearly explains the situation to the patient that they will have to be cancelled until tomorrow as there is a life threatening operation that needs to happen before them				
Apologises • Apologises for the situation but does not place or accept blame • The candidate should be empathic, but remain firm that the operation cannot be done today and not make false promises.				
ICE • The candidate explores the patients concerns and re-assures that the operation will be re-scheduled				
Answer Questions and Closes • Answers the patient's questions • Summarise, offer support/discussion with senior if necessary and make a plan				

COMMUNICATION

Communication Skills	Mark (0-4)			
Introduction • Uses appropriate opening/introductions and establishes purpose of the interview. • Ascertains what the patient already knows				
Language • Uses technical/non-technical language appropriately, accurately and with fluency. • Adapts language/behaviour as needed and adjusts style of questioning (open/closed) as appropriate, with good rapport and appropriate body language. • Clear communication.				
Listening and Rapport • Establishes relationship of respect with patient. • Demonstrates active listening. • Addresses patient's concerns and reassures				
Empathy • Demonstrates empathy and responds appropriately to patient's concerns and questions. • Aware of patient's frustration				
Closure and Timing • Adequate closure of interview. • Closes within allocated time.				

Professionalism	Mark (0-4)			
Overall Conduct • Good time management. • Demonstrates strategic and tactical planning ability. • Is sympathetic to this patient's problems. • Explains that the cancellation is no one's fault but apologises for the situation				

Follow On Questions

If the patient with appendicitis was very unwell what could be an alternative possible strategy?

Perform the appendicectomy after the AAA repair even if it is after midnight as the patient is sick and cannot wait until tomorrow morning

What are the NCEPOD codes used when booking an emergency case?

NCEPOD 1 Emergency	Immediate life-saving operation, resuscitation simultaneous with surgical treatment (e.g. trauma, ruptured AAA)	Within 1 hour
NCEPOD 1a	Operation not required immediately but must take place as soon as possible (e.g. intra-abdominal sepsis, open fracture)	Within 6 hours
NCEPOD 2 Urgent	Operation as soon as possible after resuscitation (e.g. irreducible hernia, intestinal obstruction)	Within 24hours
NCEPOD 2a	Time critical surgery (e.g. required to maximize functional recovery such as nerve or tendon repair)	Usually within 72 hours
NCEPOD 3 Scheduled	An early operation but not immediately life-saving (e.g. malignancy)	Within 3 weeks
NCEPOD 4 Elective	Operation at a time to suit both patient and surgeon (e.g. joint replacement)	At a time to suit the patient and surgeon

Examiner's Overall Assessment		
Pass	Fail	Borderline

COMMUNICATION

1.5 | Claudication History

 Candidate Briefing

You are the SHO in vascular outpatients and have been asked to see a new GP referral. Mr/Mrs Green is a 52-year-old gentleman whose letter states he has been getting increasing pain in his legs on walking. Please take an appropriate history.

 Actor Briefing

You are 52-year-old Mr/Mrs Green, you have been referred after seeing your GP with worsening pain over the last 3 months.

The pain is mainly in your right thigh and now has progressed to the right buttock as well. It is a cramping pain that stops you walking. You make it go away by stopping until the pain has gone and then carry on walking but it always comes back.

You could walk 5 miles easily before but now you struggle do half a mile before the pain is unbearable. There is no pain at rest or at night.

You have had no leg ulcers or wounds.
No previous leg or back trauma. No urinary or faecal incontinence.
You smoke 15 cigarettes a day and have done all your life and drink a few pints at the weekend.

PMH: Type 2 diabetes, hypertension

DH: NKDA. Metformin 1g BD, Ramipril 5mg OD, Paracetamol 1g PRN

SH: You live with your wife, still drive, independent of ADLs, and work as a postman.

Systems review: Your diabetes is fairly well controlled now on metformin. No other diabetic complications present.
No weight loss, change in bowel habit or urinary symptoms.

ICE: You think it is probably just "old age" but it is starting to get in the way of work which worries you. You just need the pain to go away.

COMMUNICATION

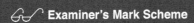

Examiner's Mark Scheme

History Taking	Mark (0-4)			
Introduction • Introduces self to patient and explains role				
Presenting Complaint • Accurately takes a pain description. • Differentiates claudication from critical limb ischaemia (rest pain, night pain and tissue loss).				
Vascular Risk Factors • Asks for vascular risk factors: hypertension, diabetes, smoking, previous stroke/MI.				
PMH, DH, SH and systems review • Has a systematic approach. • Elicits vascular risk factors as above				
ICE • Addresses the patient's ideas, concerns and expectations.				

Presenting The History	Mark (0-4)			
Summarises Key Points • Presents a well-structured history.				

Clinical Knowledge	Mark (0-4)			
Understands Vascular Symptoms • Accurately describes key clinical symptoms of intermittent claudication. • Understands key clinical signs.				
Suggests Appropriate Management • Proposes further tests such as ABPIs, duplex ultrasound • Considers risk factor reduction and level of occlusion • Considers further follow up to assess progression				

COMMUNICATION

Communication Skills	Mark (0-4)			
Introduction • Uses appropriate opening/introductions and establishes purpose of the interview. • Ascertains what the patient already knows				
Language • Uses technical/non-technical language appropriately, accurately and with fluency. • Adapts language/behaviour as needed and adjusts style of questioning (open/closed) as appropriate, with good rapport and appropriate body language. • Clear communication.				
Listening and Rapport • Establishes relationship of respect with patient. • Demonstrates active listening. • Addresses patient's concerns and expectations • Takes a comprehensive history from the patient				
Empathy • Demonstrates empathy and responds appropriately to patient's concerns and questions.				
Closure and Timing • Adequate closure of interview. • Closes within allocated time.				

Professionalism	Mark (0-4)			
Overall Conduct • Plans ahead, identifying requirements and prioritizing accordingly. • Good time management. • Appreciates need for further investigation • Is sympathetic to this patient's problems.				

Follow On Questions

How do you wish to proceed?

ABPIs today in clinic, arterial duplex as an outpatient, FBC, U+E, HbA1c, cholesterol and clotting.

What vessels are you concerned are involved based on his pain history?

Right common/external iliac and superficial femoral artery.

What lifestyle advice and medications would be of benefit?

Diabetic control with HbA1c up to date, regular exercise through the pain, smoking cessation. Start an anti-platelet and a statin, if no contra-indications.

Examiner's Overall Assessment		
Pass	Fail	Borderline

COMMUNICATION

TOP TIPS

✚ It is crucial to rule out critical limb ischaemia here as this changes the management plan.

✚ Focus the history on vascular risk factors in the limited time given in the station.

1.6 | Colorectal History

 Candidate Briefing

Mr/Mrs Halden is a 65 year-old normally fit and well patient who has presented to surgical outpatients clinic with a history of a change in bowel habit. Please take a history from him/her, then answer the examiner's questions

---

 Actor Briefing

You are Mr/Mrs Halden, are 65 years-old and normally fit and well.

In the last 4 or 5 months you have noticed that you are intermittently constipated. You do occasionally have some diarrhoea but less often. You have occasionally noticed some bright red blood on the toilet paper.

You think you have maybe lost a bit of weight over the same period – you are reasonably active so think it may be just due to that. You have lost about half a stone. Your energy levels are normal.

You have no abdominal pain that you have noticed. You are not nauseated. You have no urinary or gynaecological symptoms.

PMH: Appendicectomy aged 15.

DH: Allergic to penicillin. No regular medications.

FH: Mother has diverticular disease. Father died of heart attack aged 66.

SH: You drink 3-4 glasses of wine a week. You are an ex-smoker – you smoked 10 cigarettes a day for about 10 years, quitting 40 years ago. You are a retired secretary. You live independently with your husband/wife.

Systems Review: Nil else of note

ICE: You find it very embarassing talking about your problem and are worried because your father died aged 66.

✍ Examiner's Mark Scheme

History Taking	Mark (0-4)			
Introduction • Introduces self to patient and explains role				
Presenting Complaint • Elicits necessary information from patient • Accurately identifies and interprets key clinical features • Elicits change in bowel habit over 5 months.				
Change in Bowel Habit Red Flags • Elicits red flag symptoms: unintended weight loss, PR bleeding				
PMH, DH, SH and systems review • Has a systematic approach. • Elicits bowel risk factors as above • Satisfactory general assessment of patient				
ICE • Addresses patient's ideas, concerns and expectations				

Presenting The History	Mark (0-4)			
Summarises Key Points • Presents a well-structured history.				

Clinical Knowledge	Mark (0-4)			
Understands Bowel Symptoms • Key features are bowel habit change, weight loss, ex-smoker, PR bleed • Accurately describes key clinical symptoms. • Understands key clinical signs.				
Suggests Appropriate Management • Able to use history to suggest a sensible management plan. • Proposes further tests such as PR, flexisig/colonoscopy • Considers differential including haemorrhoids, polyp, diverticular disease, cancer				

COMMUNICATION

COMMUNICATION

Communication Skills	Mark (0-4)			
Introduction • Uses appropriate opening/introductions and establishes purpose of the interview. • Ascertains what the patient already knows				
Language • Uses technical/non-technical language appropriately, accurately and with fluency. • Adapts language/behaviour as needed and adjusts style of questioning (open/closed) as appropriate, with good rapport and appropriate body language. • Clear communication.				
Listening and Rapport • Establishes relationship of respect with patient. • Demonstrates active listening. • Addresses patient's concerns and expectations • Takes a comprehensive history from the patient				
Empathy • Demonstrates empathy and responds appropriately to patient's concerns and questions. • Does not worry patient excessively with possible diagnosis at this stage – need to await results of investigations. • Appreciates that patient finds it difficult talking about bowel problems				
Closure and Timing • Adequate closure of interview. • Closes within allocated time.				

Professionalism	Mark (0-4)			
Overall Conduct • Good time management. • Appreciates need for further investigation • Is sympathetic to this patient's problems.				

COMMUNICATION

Follow On Questions

What are some risk factors for colorectal cancer?

Congenital: positive family history, familial cancer syndromes eg FAP or HNPCC
Acquired: IBD, high fat/red meat diet, smoking, alcohol use, obesity, physical inactivity

What is the adenoma-carcinoma sequence?

This describes the succession of mutations that activate oncogenes and inactivate tumour suppressor genes, causing a progressive increase in dysplasia of a cell line until malignancy is established. Genes involved include APC, p53, TGF-beta and DCC (deleted in colorectal cancer).

What is the prognosis of colorectal cancer?

Overall 5 year survival is around 60%. Prognosis of course varies with stage and grade. T1 and T2 tumours have 5 year survival of around 90%. Spread to nodes reduces this to 40% and distant metastases to 5%.

Examiner's Overall Assessment		
Pass	Fail	Borderline

TOP TIPS

 Remember to screen for red flags early in the history.

 When suggesting a management plan remember to mention that you want to exclude something serious like a cancer so that the patient is prepared should this be the case.

1.7 | Confused Patient

 Candidate Briefing

Mr/Mrs Arnold is a 78 year-old patient who has presented to the surgical admissions lounge prior to a planned laparoscopic cholecystectomy. The nurses have asked you to see her and go through the consent process. Please see this patient, discuss the procedure and then answer the examiner's questions.

 Actor Briefing

You are Mr/Mrs Arnold. You come across as pleasant but confused.

You know your name and date of birth but cannot answer any other questions on the abbreviated mental test score (AMTS).

You are not sure why you are here – your daughter dropped you off. You think she has gone to the shops then is coming back soon to pick you up and go to the theatre.

You can answer some questions sensibly but you should come across as muddled.

The candidate should have a discussion with you about the operation but should recognise that you are confused and assess your mental state.

👓 Examiner's Mark Scheme

History Taking	Mark (0-4)			
Introduction • Introduces self and checks who the patient is • Starts with an open question such as "why are you here today?"				
Recognition of Confusion • Recognises early on that the patient is confused and doesn't have capacity to consent for the procedure				
Mini-Mental Test Scoring • Assesses the patient's capacity using the abbreviated mental test:				
- Age				
- Time				
- Address for recall at the end of the test "42 West Street"				
- Year				
- Name of this place				
- Identification of two persons (doctor, nurse etc)				
- Date of birth				
- Year of First World War				
- Name of the present Monarch				
- Count backwards from 20 to 1				
- Recalls address correctly?				
PMH, DH, SH and systems review • Attempts to establish family/NOK to contact. • Performs systems enquiry to ellict any symptoms that may have led to an acute confusional state				

COMMUNICATION

Clinical Knowledge	Mark (0-4)			
Identifies Key Issues • Accurately describes key clinical issues including a lack of capacity to consent, cancelling operation today (elective, non-life saving), informing the team and theatres, informing the family, organizing follow-up including possible admission if acutely unwell.				
Identifies and Assesses Confusion • Understands key clinical signs. • Calculates an AMT score out of 10 • Able to describe how to assess capacity and take valid informed consent.				

Communication Skills	Mark (0-4)			
Language • Uses technical/non-technical language appropriately, accurately and with fluency. • Adapts language/behaviour as needed and adjusts style of questioning (open/closed) as appropriate, with good rapport and appropriate body language. • Clear communication.				
Listening and Rapport • Appreciates confusion • Uses closed questions to elicits symptoms suggestive of an acute illness- chest/abdominal pain, cough, vomiting etc.				
Empathy • Demonstrates appreciation of confused state				
Closure and Timing • Adequate closure of interview. • Closes within allocated time.				

Professionalism	Mark (0-4)			
Overall Conduct • Good time management. • Appreciates need for further investigation • Is sympathetic to this patient's problems.				

COMMUNICATION

Follow On Questions

Having spoken to this patient, what is your impression? Can you consent her for this procedure?

Candidate should say no and outline their reasons why

What is capacity?

Capacity requires the patient to fulfill 4 criteria – they must be able to understand, retain, evaluate and communicate a decision.

Do you believe this patient has capacity? Why/why not?

It should be evident that the patient lacks capacity as she is not orientated and lacks the ability to understand, retain or evaluate the information given.

What is necessary for a patient to give an informed consent?

There are three necessary criteria – disclosure, capacity and voluntariness. Disclosure requires the patient to be in possession of all the facts relating to the decision. Capacity is as above. Voluntariness refers to patient not being encouraged or coerced into any one decision.

Examiner's Overall Assessment		
Pass	Fail	Borderline

COMMUNICATION

TOP TIPS

➕ Consent form 1 is used for adults with capacity undergoing a procedure under general anaesthetic, local anaesthetic or sedation

➕ Consent form 2 is used for paediatric patients

➕ Consent form 3 is used for procedures that are undertaken without impairment of consciousness, such as those under local anaesthetic

➕ Consent form 4 is used where a patient is found to lack capacity and so a procedure is being undertaken in their best interests

1.8 | Epigastric Pain History

 Candidate Briefing

Mr/Mrs Crawford is a 58 year old who has been referred to the surgical outpatient clinic by his GP with a 6-week history of burning epigastric discomfort. Please take a history from them, and then answer the examiner's questions.

 Actor Briefing

You are Mr/Mrs Crawford. You have had a pain in the centre of your stomach for the last 6 or 8 weeks. It also goes into your chest a bit and also through to your back but does not goes anywhere else. It feels like a burning pain and stabbing at its worst. It is worst not long after you have eaten. Nothing seems to make it better particularly. It is present all the time and doesn't change particularly unless you have something to eat.

You have had no change in your bowel habit, no urinary symptoms and no hot or cold sweats. You have no history of abdominal problems and you have never really had symptoms like this before. You have had heartburn on occasion, but it has always gone away.

Only if asked specifically by the candidate:

You have lost about half a stone over the same time – you have not been trying to particularly as you have never been overweight.

More recently you think occasionally you feel food sticking for a short time very low in your chest behind your breastbone. You do not bring any food back up but you do get heartburn and acid in the back of your throat sometimes.

PMH: Hypothyroidism

DH: No allergies. Thyroxine OD, PRN paracetamol, ibuprofen and gaviscon when you get the pain

SH: You work as a cashier in a bank. You live with your partner and two children. You are independently mobile and healthy. You have no pets. You smoke 20 cigarettes a day and have done since you were 18. You drink about 5-6 glasses of wine a week.

FH: Your father died of a heart attack aged 70, your mother is still alive and is fit and well.

Systems Review: Nil else of note

ICE: Your GP has suggested some things to try like stopping smoking, which you have struggled with. You have managed to cut down on fatty foods but this has made no difference. You would like to know what is going on – you wonder whether it might gallstones as your partner had these and had to have his gallbladder removed.

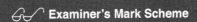 **Examiner's Mark Scheme**

History Taking	Mark (0-4)			
Introduction • Introduces self and checks who the patient is				
History Of Presenting Complaint • Elicits necessary information from patient • Accurately identifies and interprets key clinical features • Performs a thorough pain history				
Upper GI Red Flags • Elicits red flag symptoms of an upper GI malignancy: unintended weight loss, swallowing difficulties, reflux				
PMH, DH, SH and systems review • Has a systematic approach. • Satisfactory general assessment of patient and social circumstances				
ICE • Addresses patient's ideas, concerns and expectations				

Presenting The History	Mark (0-4)			
Summarises Key Issues • Presents a well-structured history.				

Clinical Knowledge	Mark (0-4)			
Identifies Key Upper GI Issues • Key features are weight loss, smoker, swallowing difficulties • Accurately describes key clinical symptoms. • Understands key clinical signs.				
Management Plan • Suggests differential diagnosis: peptic ulcer, gastritis, GORD, oesophageal/gastric cancer • Able to use history to suggest a sensible management plan. • Bloods, OGD, PPI therapy				

COMMUNICATION

Communication Skills	Mark (0-4)			
Introduction • Uses appropriate opening/introductions and establishes purpose of the interview. • Ascertains what the patient already knows				
Language • Uses technical/non-technical language appropriately, accurately and with fluency. • Adapts language/behaviour as needed and adjusts style of questioning (open/closed) as appropriate, with good rapport and appropriate body language. • Clear communication.				
Listening and Rapport • Establishes relationship of respect with patient. • Demonstrates active listening. • Addresses patient's concerns and expectations • Takes a comprehensive history from the patient				
Empathy • Demonstrates empathy and responds appropriately to patient's concerns and questions. • Does not worry patient excessively with possible diagnosis at this stage – need to await results of investigations.				
Closure and Timing • Adequate closure of interview. • Closes within allocated time.				

Professionalism	Mark (0-4)			
Overall Conduct • Good time management. • Appreciates need for further investigation • Is sympathetic to this patient's problems.				

Follow On Questions

What are your differential diagnoses?

The main concern is for upper GI malignancy . Other differentials would include severe reflux, gallstones or pharyngeal pouch, peptic ulcer, pancreatitis, pancreatic malignancy, angina/ischaemic heart disease

How would you investigate this patient?

Urgent 2 week wait OGD.
Routine bloods including FBC, U+E, LFT, lipase, CA 19-9
An abdomen ultrasound would also be a useful first imaging investigation.
If malignancy is identified or suspected from these first investigations, a CT chest, abdomen and pelvis should be performed looking for metastatic spread.

Examiner's Overall Assessment		
Pass	Fail	Borderline

COMMUNICATION

TOP TIPS

➕ In this scenario the actor has been briefed to only reveal certain red flag symptoms if specifically asked. Ensure you know what these are.

➕ The patient thinks it might be due to gallstones but hasn't considered anything more serious. Make sure you discuss all possibilities and clearly outline a management and follow up plan.

COMMUNICATION

1.9 | Erectile Dysfunction History

 Candidate Briefing

You are an SHO in the urology clinic. Mr T is a 50-year-old builder who has come to discuss problems he is having maintaining an erection. Please take a history from him, then present to the examiner & answer their questions.

 Actor Briefing

You are a 50-year-old builder. For the past 9 months you have had trouble both obtaining & maintaining an erection during sexual intercourse with your wife. The problem is worsening, now within a few minutes you have to stop, you haven't tried anything to improve it as you are not sure what the problem is. Your wife has also begun to notice. You have never had the problem before.

PMH: Angina diagnosed by cardiologist 2 years ago
You can walk a good few miles and still work but you are now mostly in the office. You have noticed your exercise tolerance is becoming more limited. You think you had a normal ECHO last year and have never had an angiogram.
Hypertension.
No previous heart attacks, strokes or problems with peripheral vessels, no diabetes.

DH: Lisinopril 10mg OD, Simvastatin 40mg OD, Bisoprolol 1.25mg OD, GTN spray PRN

SH: You live with your wife and 2 children, stable work & home, no financial concerns, no extra-marital affairs

Systems Review: NAD

ICE: You are anxious that this will affect your marriage

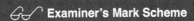

Examiner's Mark Scheme

History Taking	Mark (0-4)			
Introduction • Introduces self and checks who the patient is				
History Of Presenting Complaint • Elicits necessary information from patient • Accurately identifies and interprets key clinical features				
Erectile Dysfunction Specifics • Performs a thorough symptom history- is it maintaining an erection that is difficult or getting one? Do they have spontaneous erections still particularly nocturnal erections? • Respectfully enquires about social situation such as sexual partners and potential external stressors that patient may have such as loss of job or financial worries				
PMH, DH, SH and systems review • Has a systematic approach. • Satisfactory general assessment of patient and social circumstances				
ICE • Addresses patient's ideas, concerns and expectations				

Presenting The History	Mark (0-4)		
Summarises Key Issues • Presents a well-structured history.			

Clinical Knowledge	Mark (0-4)		
Identifies Key Erectile Dysfunction Issues • Key features are difficulties maintaining an erection, ischaemic heart disease and that the patient is married with no external stressors • Understands key clinical signs to help differentiate between a psychogenic and organic cause for erectile dysfunction, such as nocturnal erections suggest a psychogenic cause			

COMMUNICATION

COMMUNICATION

Communication Skills	Mark (0-4)			
Introduction • Uses appropriate opening/introductions and establishes purpose of the interview. • Ascertains what the patient already knows				
Language • Uses technical/non-technical language appropriately, accurately and with fluency. • Adapts language/behaviour as needed and adjusts style of questioning (open/closed) as appropriate, with good rapport and appropriate body language. • Clear communication.				
Listening and Rapport • Establishes relationship of respect with patient. • Demonstrates active listening. • Addresses patient's concerns and expectations • Takes a comprehensive history from the patient				
Empathy • Demonstrates empathy and responds appropriately to patient's concerns and questions. • Deals sensitively with personal questions and sexual history				
Closure and Timing • Adequate closure of interview. • Closes within allocated time.				

Professionalism	Mark (0-4)			
Overall Conduct • Good time management. • Appreciates the potential embarrassing and very personal nature of this complaint and behaves accordingly • Is sympathetic to this patient's problems.				

Follow On Questions

What is erectile dysfunction?

Defined as the persistent inability to obtain & maintain an erection sufficient for sexual intercourse. Prevalence 5% aged 40 to 15% aged 70.

How can it be classified?

Psychogenic or organic. Relative incidences of each are about 50:50.

What are the major organic causes?

Vascular disease, neurogenic (for example, spinal injury, MS), trauma (pelvic fracture/surgery), drugs (anti-hypertensives, anti-depressants, alcohol), hypogonadism (pituitary or gonadal), or chronic illness

What investigations are useful for assessment?

Examination of peripheral pulses, external genitalia & digital rectal examination. Urinanalysis for glucose. Serum testosterone and prolactin, looking for hypogonadism

Examiner's Overall Assessment		
Pass	Fail	Borderline

COMMUNICATION

TOP TIPS

➕ Erectile dysfunction can be psychogenic or organic. Target your history at finding out what the underlying cause might be.

➕ Prevalence of ED is 5% aged 40 to 15% aged 70.

➕ A large part of this station is ensuring you take a respectful, careful history.

1.10 Difficulty Swallowing History

 Candidate Briefing

You are the surgical SHO on call. James, a 14-year-old boy , presents with difficulty swallowing. His mother accompanies him. Please take a focused history and then answer the examiners questions.

 Actor Briefing

You are James, a 14-year-old boy who has been finding it painful to swallow. You are coming to hospital with your mother.

You have been getting recurrent sore throats for the last 6 weeks and been given antibiotics by the OOH GP 2 weeks ago who says she saw one big tonsil. If asked you have also been suffering from nasal blockage and a weird sound to your voice. Your mum has also been saying that you have been snoring and sweating at night for the past 2 weeks. You have lost quite a bit of weight the last 6 weeks, which your mum is really worried about.

PMH: Nil, up-to-date with vaccinations

FH: Nil

DH: Nil regular, NKDA

SH: Avid footballer, meeting all developmental milestones, no perinatal issues. Parents are non-smokers

Systems Review: A mild upper abdominal ache that improves with paracetamol. No nausea or vomiting. Bowels are normal.

ICE: The GP mentioned that one of your tonsils appeared larger than the other, but didn't explain why he was referring you in to see the specialist.

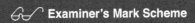

Examiner's Mark Scheme

History Taking	Mark (0-4)			
Introduction • Introduces self and checks patient identity				
History Of Presenting Complaint • Elicits necessary information from patient • Accurately identifies and interprets key clinical features: painful vs painless, solids vs liquids, associated swelling?				
Swallowing Red Flags • Accurately identifies and interprets key clinical features such as red flag symptoms. • Specific red flag symptoms to cover are night sweats and weight loss (B symptoms), dysphonia, abdominal pain, neck swelling				
PMH, DH, SH and systems review • Has a systematic approach. • Satisfactory general assessment of patient and social circumstances				
ICE • Addresses patient's ideas, concerns and expectations				

Presenting The History	Mark (0-4)			
Summarises Key Issues • Presents a well-structured history.				

Clinical Knowledge	Mark (0-4)			
Identifies Key Swallowing Issues • Accurately describes key clinical symptoms such as weight loss, recurrent infections and enlarged tonsil. • Appreciates the potential seriousness of the history- this may be a first presentation of lymphoma in a child.				
Differential Diagnosis • Differentials would be infectious mononucleosis (Epstein-Barr infection), squamous-cell carcinoma, sarcoidosis, lymphoma.				

COMMUNICATION

COMMUNICATION

Communication Skills	Mark (0-4)			
Introduction • Uses appropriate opening/introductions and establishes purpose of the interview. • Ascertains what the patient already knows • Aims to communicate with the child primarily but questions the mother when needed				
Language • Uses technical/non-technical language appropriately, accurately and with fluency. • Adapts language/behaviour as needed and adjusts style of questioning (open/closed) as appropriate, with good rapport and appropriate body language. • Clear communication.				
Listening and Rapport • Establishes relationship of respect with patient. • Demonstrates active listening. • Addresses patient's concerns and expectations • Takes a comprehensive history from the patient				
Empathy • Demonstrates empathy and responds appropriately to patient's concerns and questions. • Explains further investigations required				
Closure and Timing • Adequate closure of interview. • Closes within allocated time.				

Professionalism	Mark (0-4)			
Overall Conduct • Good time management. • Communicates with both child and relatives. • Is sympathetic to this patient's problems.				

Follow On Questions

What are your differential diagnoses from this history?

Tonsillar non-Hodgkin's lymphoma (NHL), infectious mononucleosis (Epstein-Barr infection), squamous-cell carcinoma and sarcoidosis.

Histologically, how can Hodgkin's lymphoma (HL) be differentiated from NHL?

The presence of Reed Sternberg cells in HL is diagnostic.

Based on the history, how would you examine this patient?

Full head, neck and oral cavity examination, abdominal, groin and axillary examination for organomegaly and other lymphadenopathy.

What would your first line investigation be for this patient?

Ultrasound (USS) neck and abdomen, with fine needle aspiration (FNA) of any neck lumps or excision biopsy.

Examiner's Overall Assessment		
Pass	Fail	Borderline

TOP TIPS

➕ NHL has generally a fair prognosis, up to around 80% at 5 years, dependant on stage, grade and cell line. 75% of patients with tonsillar NHL will have localised disease on presentation.

➕ USS is followed by FNA/excisional biopsy for histology, staging scans *(CT/MRI/PET)* and then discussion at the lymphoma MDT.

➕ Treatment depends on the stage and MDT discussion. Options include radiotherapy, chemotherapy, chemo-radiotherapy, radio-immunotherapy and surgery *(the latter reserved for histological diagnoses requiring de-bulking only.)*

1.11 | Urinary Tract Symptoms History

 Candidate Briefing

You are the general surgical SHO on call. Mr T is a 65-year-old who has been referred by ED with urinary retention. Please take an appropriate history from him, then present to the examiner.

 Actor Briefing

You are 65 years old. You have not passed urine for 4 days, despite drinking lots of water to help. You are beginning to feel some abdominal discomfort. Additionally you have felt hot and sweaty in the last 24 hours with some shivering episodes.

You have had some problems urinating for over 2 years. Initially it was a delay on starting to urinate which has progressed rapidly over the last few months to a slow stream with a feeling of not completely emptying your bladder. If asked, you have also noticed blood in your urine. You have ignored it as you hoped it was nothing worrying. You have had no burning on passing urine, no dribbling, no sudden need to pass urine, no need to get up at night to urinate and no episodes of incontinence.
You have not lost any weight, have no pain and no history of renal stones.

You haven't seen your GP because you don't want to waste their time and you are too busy with work recently to fit in an appointment.

PMH: Nil

DH: Nil, NKDA

SH: Lives with wife, accountant

Systems Review: NAD

COMMUNICATION

✐ Examiner's Mark Scheme

History Taking	Mark (0-4)			
Introduction • Introduces self and checks patient identity				
History Of Presenting Complaint • Elicits necessary information from patient • Accurately identifies and interprets key clinical features of chronic bladder outflow obstruction but with an acute infective history				
Micturition Red Flags • Thorough micturition history covering initiation, stream, incomplete voiding, dysuria and haematuria • Elicits red flag symptoms of possible malignancy- haematuria				
PMH, DH, SH and systems review • Has a systematic approach. • Satisfactory general assessment of patient and social circumstances				
ICE • Addresses patient's ideas, concerns and expectations				

Presenting The History	Mark (0-4)			
Summarises Key Issues • Presents a well-structured history.				

Clinical Knowledge	Mark (0-4)			
Identifies Key Clinical Issues • Key features are mentioned such as rigors, increasing difficulty urinating and haematuria • Understands key clinical signs such as the patient is suffering from a urinary tract infection which has led to acute retention and sepsis.				

COMMUNICATION

Communication Skills	Mark (0-4)			
Introduction • Uses appropriate opening/introductions and establishes purpose of the interview. • Ascertains what the patient already knows				
Language • Uses technical/non-technical language appropriately, accurately and with fluency. • Adapts language/behaviour as needed and adjusts style of questioning (open/closed) as appropriate, with good rapport and appropriate body language. • Clear communication.				
Listening and Rapport • Establishes relationship of respect with patient. • Demonstrates active listening. • Addresses patient's concerns and expectations • Takes a comprehensive history from the patient				
Empathy • Demonstrates empathy and responds appropriately to patient's concerns and questions. • Explains further investigations required				
Closure and Timing • Adequate closure of interview. • Closes within allocated time.				

Professionalism	Mark (0-4)			
Overall Conduct • Good time management. • Communicates sensitively • Is sympathetic to this patient's problems.				

Follow On Questions

What is your differential diagnosis in this case?

This is chronic bladder outflow obstruction.
Benign: benign prostatic hyperplasia, urethral stricture, bladder calculus, neuropathic bladder dysfunction.
Neoplastic: prostate cancer, bladder cancer

What is PSA?

Prostate-specific antigen. This has an age-specific range. Highly sensitive for prostate cancer but low specificity.

What conditions raise this marker?

Prostate disease, acute urinary retention, UTI, after DRE (so best taken before).

What condition is suspected with a high serum PSA level?

Prostate cancer

Please name and briefly describe a prognostic scoring system for prostate cancer

The Gleason grading system. A numerical score is given: 2 (well differentiated tumours) to 10 (least differentiated tumours). The score is based on adverse features found on histology, marked using specific 'Gleason patterns'. A calculation using these patterns gives the overall score.

Examiner's Overall Assessment		
Pass	Fail	Borderline

TOP TIPS

You may be asked to briefly describe the Gleason system. It is a numerical score: 2 *(well differentiated tumours)* to 10 *(least differentiated tumours)*. The score is based on adverse features found on histology, marked using specific 'Gleason patterns'. A calculation using these patterns gives the overall score.

COMMUNICATION

1.12 | Parental Consent

COMMUNICATION

 Candidate Briefing

You are the general surgical SHO on call. Your team has admitted Paul, an 8-year-old boy who has suspected perforated appendicitis. He is currently on the ward, and is the priority for theatres. Your registrar has spoken to Paul and his father, who has signed a parental consent form. Paul is tachycardic and in pain but is otherwise stable. He came in with his father and is otherwise a well child with no past medical history.

His mother has arrived and wants to speak to you about what is happening. She is very worried. She is divorced from Paul's father. Your registrar is busy in theatre.

Please speak to Paul's mother and answer her questions. You do not need to take a full history.

 Actor Briefing

You are Jane Wallace, the mother of Paul.

You were at work today and were called by your ex-husband from A&E about your eldest son an hour ago. He explained that he is in a lot of pain and needed to come into hospital. He then called saying Paul needs an operation on his abdomen. You rushed straight in and have seen Paul on the ward briefly. You know nothing else.

You are extremely worried, bordering on panic. You want to know what has happened to your son, why he is so unwell, and what is the plan.

You don't understand hospital jargon.

You and Paul's father divorced 3 years ago and do not speak. His name is on Paul's birth certificate.

Your specific concerns are:
• What is wrong with your son?
• How unwell is he and is there a possibility he may die?
• What are the surgeons planning on doing in the operation?
• What will happen afterwards?
• You know this needs written consent- who has given that?
• You agree with Paul's father signing the consent form but you would like to go through the specific of the procedure including the risks.

COMMUNICATION

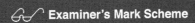 **Examiner's Mark Scheme**

Consent	Mark (0-4)			
Introduction • Introduces self and checks patient identity • Candidate checks what the mother's understanding of the situation is				
Explanation • Proceeds to explain what is wrong with her son and the plan as made by the registrar • Checks the relatives understanding of what is being discussed • Recognises this is a difficult discussion with a worried parent • The candidate should discuss the consent form for the operation with the mother				
Establishing Consent • Can explain to the mother about who can consent for Paul to have his operation using current guidance				

Clinical Knowledge	Mark (0-4)			
Consenting a Child • If a child lacks the capacity to consent, a doctor can ask the parents. • Usually one parent is enough. For young people who lack capacity the law differs across the UK. In England and Wales, parents can consent for treatment and investigations in the young person's best interests, or the medical team can make decisions without parental consent. In Scotland young people who lack capacity are managed as adults who lack capacity • The term 'parents' means those who have parental responsibility in law for a child or young person. The mother and the father who was married to the mother at the time of birth have automatic parental responsibility. • This also applies to an unmarried father who has their name on the child's birth certificate registered after December 2003 in England and Wales (different dates apply for Scotland and Northern Ireland).				

• Divorce does not change parental responsibility. An unmarried father whose child was registered before the date above, or who is not named on the birth certificate does not have automatic parental responsibility, although he can apply for it. • The same can be done by step-parents and civil partners. Adoption removes parental responsibility from the parents, and a court order can restrict it. A local authority can share responsibility if the child is taken into care. • Patients under the age of 18 are young people according the UK law. • Understands how to obtain valid consent for paediatric patients				

Communication Skills	Mark (0-4)			
Language • Uses technical/non-technical language appropriately, accurately and with fluency. • Adapts language/behaviour as needed and adjusts style of questioning (open/closed) as appropriate, with good rapport and appropriate body language. • Clear communication.				
Listening and Rapport • Establishes relationship of respect with patient. • Demonstrates active listening. • Addresses patient's concerns and expectations				
Empathy • Demonstrates empathy and responds appropriately to patient's concerns and questions.				
Closure and Timing • Adequate closure of interview. • Closes within allocated time.				

Professionalism	Mark (0-4)			
Overall Conduct • Good time management. • Communicates with both child and relatives. • Is sympathetic to this patient's problems.				

Follow On Questions

Where could you find advice on consenting paediatric patients?

GMC guidance on the care of children is set out in the document: '0-18 years: guidance for all doctors'.

What if a child refuses a procedure who is deemed to have capacity to do so?

A child can consent to a procedure if they are deemed Gilllick competent however they cannot refuse any treatment that is deemed in their best interest.

What if a child deemed competent asks you not to inform their parents?

The involvement of a young person's family and carers is important, irrespective of a child's capacity to consent. If a child can decide on their own care, they should be encouraged to involve their parents or carers at all times however doctor patient confidentiality rules must be adhered to also.

Examiner's Overall Assessment		
Pass	Fail	Borderline

COMMUNICATION

TOP TIPS

➕ At 16 and over, it is legally presumed that a young person has the ability to make their own decisions about their medical care.

➕ Younger children may have the capacity to consent to their care, if they are competent to do so.

➕ Competency is not presumed, but can be proven by assessing the child's ability to understand, weigh up, recall and communicate their decision. Each individual child will be different.

➕ Several factors will affect their capacity, including the complexity of the decision in front of them, their physical health and emotional development.

1.13 | Pre-Operative Assessment History

 Candidate Briefing

You are asked to attend pre-operative assessment clinic to see a patient who has been booked for an anterior resection for a high rectal cancer. Please take an appropriate history to assess their fitness for surgery, and then answer the examiner's questions.

 Actor Briefing

You are Mr/Mrs J Smith, a 63-year-old who presented 6 weeks ago with a 6 month history of change in bowel habit and sensation of incomplete empty-ing. You underwent flexible sigmoidoscopy and a CT and then MRI scan, and you know you have a tumour in your rectum that needs a major opera-tion.

PMH: Diabetes, COPD , Hypothyroidism, Hypertension, Appendicectomy aged 11

DH: Allergic to penicillin, Metformin, glicazide, salbutamol, symbicort, thyroxin, ramipril

SH: Ex-smoker, occasional alcohol – 4units/week.
You can walk about 100-150 yards on the flat before you need to catch your breath. You need one rest on a flight of stairs.
You live with your husband.

Systems Review: You can walk about 100-150 yards on the flat before you need to catch your breath. You need one rest on a flight of stairs.

ICE: You are worried about the magnitude of the operation but know it needs to be done. You ask whether it is possible to have it done under spi-nal as you don't like the thought of being asleep.

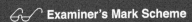

Examiner's Mark Scheme

History Taking	Mark (0-4)			
Introduction • Introduces self and checks patient identity				
Understanding and Screening • Finds out what the patient knows so far • "Why are you here today? What procedure are you having done and why?" • Clearly explains this is a pre-operative assessment to ensure the patient is as fit as possible for the procedure and has everything they need done before the day of surgery to hopefully avoid the operation being cancelled				
PMH, DH, SH and systems review • Generally the candidate will lead the interview with some closed questions following the initial discussion • Covers past medical history, particularly asking about common surgical risk factors such as ischaemic heart disease, MI in the last 6 months, diabetes, inhaler use, general fitness • Assesses the patient's social situation "Who is at home with you?", "Do you require any home help?"				
ICE • Addresses patient's ideas, concerns and expectations • Answers the patient's concerns				

Presenting The History	Mark (0-4)			
Summarises Key Issues • Summarises what will happen next "You will be contacted if there are any problems with any of the tests that need addressing before the operation"				

COMMUNICATION

COMMUNICATION

Communication Skills	Mark (0-4)			
Introduction • Uses appropriate opening/introductions and establishes purpose of the interview. • Ascertains what the patient already knows				
Language • Uses technical/non-technical language appropriately, accurately and with fluency. • Adapts language/behaviour as needed and adjusts style of questioning (open/closed) as appropriate, with good rapport and appropriate body language. • Clear communication.				
Listening and Rapport • Establishes relationship of respect with patient. • Demonstrates active listening. • Addresses patient's concerns and expectations • Takes a comprehensive history from the patient				
Empathy • Demonstrates empathy and responds appropriately to patient's concerns and questions. • Explains further investigations required				
Closure and Timing • Adequate closure of interview. • Closes within allocated time.				

Professionalism	Mark (0-4)			
Overall Conduct • Good time management. • Communicates sensitively • Is sympathetic to this patient's problems.				

Follow On Questions

What are the issues here regarding this patient's surgical fitness?

Multiple comorbidities, including diabetes, hypertension and COPD
Exercise tolerance is reduced.
All these factors increase surgical risk.

What severity of surgery is this?

This is grade 4 (major +) as it involves colonic resection.

How should the patient's peri-operative diabetes be managed?

The patient is on medication only for their diabetes. They do not necessarily need a sliding scale if the blood glucose levels are well controlled but they will need regular blood glucose monitoring.

What is enhanced recovery?

• Enhanced recovery is a systematic process encompassing the entire operative patient's journey, designed to minimize recovery time and reduce morbidity and mortality with evidence-based practices.
• The patient is optimised pre-operatively, in terms of comorbidities, nutritional status and surgical fitness.
Surgery should be as minimally invasive and atraumatic as possible.
Post-operatively, they are mobilized early. Key to this is physiotherapy and adequate pain-relief.

What other pre-operative investigations are important for this patient?

• The patient should of had a staging CT including the chest, so a CXR is not indicated unless there has been some recent change in the patient's chest symptoms.
• An ECG
• FBC, U+E, LFT, clotting and a group and save are indicated.
• A stress echo is indicated if there is a suggestion of cardiovascular disease.
• Spirometry may be useful.
There are considerable anaesthetic risk factors and so discussion and review by the anaesthetist are warranted. It may be necessary to perform some additional tests of surgical fitness, particularly a CPEX test.

Examiner's Overall Assessment		
Pass	Fail	Borderline

TOP TIPS

 Co-morbidity assessment must include severity of illness, impact on daily life, recent and acutely worsening conditions versus more stable disease

1.14 | Thyroid History

 Candidate Briefing

Mrs X is a 40-year-old normally fit and well lady who has presented to your outpatients clinic with a history of a lump in her neck. Please take her history then answer the examiners' questions

 Actor Briefing

You are Mrs X, a 40 year old normally fit and well lady who has presented to your outpatients clinic with a history of a lump in her neck. You first became aware of this several months ago and thought it was a sore throat but it has not gone away. You are not sure if it has increased in size. It is slightly painful. You have not noticed a change in voice. The lump does move when you swallow.

You have not noticed feeling hotter or colder than usual recently. You had not been trying to lose weight but people have commented that you have lost some, and your clothes are looser. You have been feeling a bit tired recently.

You have not noticed any hair or skin changes.

PMH: You had asthma as a child but nil else.

DH: NKDA, paracetamol and ibuprofen PRN.

SH: You smoke 10 cigarettes a day, drink alcohol only occasionally, work as a shop assistant.

FH: Your mother suffered with a goiter but this improved with tablets (you are not sure which).

Systems Review: You have no other systemic upset.

ICE: You are concerned that it might be cancer – what if it is? What more needs to be done?

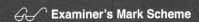

Examiner's Mark Scheme

History Taking	Mark (0-4)			
Introduction • Introduces self and checks patient identity				
Presenting Complaint • Asks questions to ellict potential thyroid symptoms such as weight gain/loss, energy levels, temperature control, tremors, palpitations • Asks questions to identify local neck lump symptoms such as any voice changes, swallowing difficulties, and shortness of breath, lump size increase or decrease, whether the lump moves with tongue movements or swallowing				
Thyroid Red Flags • Elicits red flag symptoms of a possible thyroid cancer- unintentional weight loss, lethargy, persistent neck lump				
PMH, DH, SH and systems review • Has a systematic approach. • Satisfactory general assessment of patient and social circumstances				
ICE • Addresses patient's ideas, concerns and expectations • Answers the patient's concerns				

Presenting The History	Mark (0-4)			
Summarises Key Issues • Presents a well-structured history. • Key features are weight loss and persistent neck lump • Accurately describes key clinical symptoms. • Understands key clinical signs. • Able to use history to suggest a sensible management plan.				

COMMUNICATION

COMMUNICATION

Communication Skills	Mark (0-4)			
Introduction • Uses appropriate opening/introductions and establishes purpose of the interview. • Ascertains what the patient already knows				
Language • Uses technical/non-technical language appropriately, accurately and with fluency. • Adapts language/behaviour as needed and adjusts style of questioning (open/closed) as appropriate, with good rapport and appropriate body language. • Clear communication.				
Listening and Rapport • Establishes relationship of respect with patient. • Demonstrates active listening. • Addresses patient's concerns and expectations				
Empathy • Demonstrates empathy and responds appropriately to patient's concerns and questions. • Explains further investigations required • Does not worry patient excessively with possible diagnosis at this stage – need to await results of investigations.				
Closure and Timing • Adequate closure of interview. • Closes within allocated time.				

Professionalism	Mark (0-4)			
Overall Conduct • Good time management. • Communicates sensitively • Is sympathetic to this patient's problems.				

Follow On Questions

What are your differentials?

Thyroid cancer, thyroid lymphoma, multinodular goitre.

What is the most common form of thyroid cancer? What are the others?

Papillary is most common, followed by follicular. Medullary, anaplastic and thyroid lymphoma are the others.

What are the most common routes of spread of the different thyroid cancers?

Papillary spreads via lymphatics, follicular via blood. Anaplastic spreads mainly by direct invasion.

Which carries the best and worst prognosis?

Papillary has the best prognosis. Anaplastic has the worst.

How could you investigate her?

Triple assessment. This should commence with thorough examination and bloods. You may choose to ultrasound the mass. Tissue biopsy should be undertaken by core biopsy (FNA is not useful as it cannot show histological structure, necessary for staging). A radioisotope scan may demonstrate a cold nodule. A CT may be necessary to stage if cancer is identified.

How is thyroid cancer managed?

This depends on the type, stage and grade, but can be classified into medical and surgical. Typically the surgery is total thyroidectomy, if appropriate. Remaining tissue is ablated with radioactive iodine 131. Long term TSH suppression with Thyroxine can limit further tumour growth. Nodal dissection may be performed for spread. Radiotherapy and chemotherapy are used for metastatic and unresectable disease.

Examiner's Overall Assessment		
Pass	Fail	Borderline

COMMUNICATION

TOP TIPS

+ Management of thyroid cancer depends on the type, stage and grade, but can be classified into medical and surgical. Curative surgery is in the form of total thyroidectomy, if appropriate. Remaining tissue is ablated with radioactive iodine 131. Long term TSH suppression with thyroxine can limit further tumour growth. Nodal dissection may be performed for staging. Radiotherapy and chemotherapy are used for metastatic and un-resectable disease.

2 OSCEs

2.1 | Abdominal Examination

Common Scenarios
You are unlikely to see real acute abdominal pain in the exam for obvious reasons, but common subacute causes might include:

- Bilary colic/gallstone disease
- Gastritis/peptic ulcer disease
- Chronic pancreatitis

 Candidate Briefing

Mr/Mrs B is a 45-year-old office worker who has presented with a history of intermittent epigastric pain radiating round the flanks. This settles completely between episodes. He/she has had no previous investigation, but has been referred by the GP as it is not settling down. Please examine their abdomen then answer the examiner's questions.

 Actor Briefing

You are Mr/Mrs B, a 45-year-old office worker who has presented with a history of intermittent epigastric pain radiating round the flanks.

You are tender in the epigastrium and right upper quadrant currently but with no peritonism. You are otherwise well. If the candidate asks you you are fair and overweight with a BMI of 30. You have no other stigmata of gastrointestinal/bilary disease.

Examiner's Mark Scheme

Introduction	Mark (0-4)			
The candidate should: • Wash/gel hands, explain procedure, obtain consent • Ask for a chaperone and treat the patient with dignity at all times				

OSCES

Inspection	Mark (0-4)			
• Perform a general inspection: commenting on patient and surroundings, e.g. drains, catheters, obs chart etc				
• **Hands**: commenting on nail signs, palmar signs, pulse				
• **Face**: commenting on scleral jaundice, conjunctival pallor, plethora/wasting, signs in the mouth eg ulcers, dentition				
• **Neck:** may have a cursory feel for lymph nodes particularly left supraclavicular				
• **Abdomen**: scars, shape, stomas, other stigmata eg caput medusa				

Palpation	Mark (0-4)			
• **Palpate**: all 9 regions, commenting on tenderness, masses etc.				
• **Percuss**: all 9 regions, marking out liver and spleen edges and assessing for fluid				

Auscultation	Mark (0-4)			
• **Auscultate:** for bowel sounds and bruits				

Special Tests	Mark (0-4)			
• Assess for Murphy's or Rovsing's signs • Assess for the Obturator or Psoas signs • Use patient inspiration to assess for organomegaly				

Closing	Mark (0-4)			
• Mentions would also examine hernia orifices and scrotum and do a PR • Thanks patient • Maintains patient dignity • Mentions would also examine hernia orifices and scrotum and do a PR				

Presentation	Mark (0-4)			
• Summarise their findings • Offers an appropriate differential diagnosis and management plan • Suggests appropriate inital investigations such as abdominal radiograph				

Follow On Questions

What are your differential diagnoses?

• Gallbladder pathology should be high on the list – mainly gallstones/cholecystitis
• Other differentials include gastritis/peptic ulcer, pancreatitis, renal colic, hepatitis, cancer

How will you investigate this patient?

• Bloods: FBC, U&Es, LFT, Amylase, CRP, NILS screen possibly
• Urine dip
• Abdominal ultrasound scan
• Possibly oesophago-gastro-duodenoscopy (OGD)

What are the layers of the abdominal wall through which you would go during a Kocher's incision to access the gallbladder?

• Skin, subcutaneous fat, superficial fascia, external oblique, internal oblique, transversus abdominis, transversalis fascia, pre-peritoneal fat, peritoneum

Examiner's Overall Assessment		
Pass	Fail	Borderline

TOP TIPS

 When presenting, it shows the examiners that you are safe and sensible junior surgeon if you frame your further investigations with a statement such as, *"I would wish to firstly rule out serious underlying pathology such as a neoplastic process, though I think (X, Y or Z) is the most likely cause"*. This shows that you are thinking.

2.2 | Arterial Examination

Common Scenarios

The vignette directs you towards peripheral vascular disease, but don't forget other potential similar pathologies, such as:

- Spinal stenosis
- Or neurogenic claudication.

 Candidate Briefing

Mr/Mrs X is a 68 year-old type 2 diabetic and smoker who has presented to your clinic with a history of pain in his legs. Their GP suspects intermittent claudication. Please examine him/her as you see fit, then answer the examiners' questions.

 Actor Briefing

You are Mr/Mrs X, a 68 year-old patient with pain in your legs. You get this after walking 50 yards or so, though it never used to be this bad.

You have no pain to palpation of the legs but your distal pulses should be barely palpable on examination (describe this finding to the candidate as they examine).

👓 Examiner's Mark Scheme

Introduction	Mark (0-4)			
The candidate should: • Wash/gel hands, explain procedure, obtain consent • Ask for a chaperone and treat the patient with dignity at all times				

OSCES

Inspection	Mark (0-4)			
The candidate should look for an comment on features of peripheral vascular disease, such as: • Tissue loss/ulceration • Venous guttering and hair loss • A general inspection of the patient and the bedside e.g. tar staining on fingers				

Palpation	Mark (0-4)			
• **Peripheral Pulses**: Assess for the presence of peripheral pulses – femoral, popliteal, dorsalis pedis, posterior tibial (and anterior tibial and peroneal)				
• **Temperature**: Feel the warmth of the legs, comparing side to side				
• **Perfusion**: Assess capillary refill time				
• **Aneurysms**: Palpate for abdominal aortic aneurysm				

Auscultation	Mark (0-4)			
• **Auscultate:** for bruits				

Special Tests	Mark (0-4)			
• **Buerger's test**: comment on the angle at which blood flow is compromised and the leg goes white				
• **ABPIs**: Perform or describe an ankle-brachial pressure index measurement				

Closing	Mark (0-4)			
• Thanks patient • Maintains patient dignity				

Presentation	Mark (0-4)			
• Summarise their findings • Offers an appropriate differential diagnosis and management plan				

OSCES

Presentation	Mark (0-4)			
• Suggests appropriate inital investigations such as arterial duplex				

Follow On Questions

What ABPI indicates the presence of peripheral vascular disease?

Less than 0.7

Why might an ABPI be raised greater than the normal range?

If the vessels are heavily calcified and incompressible, for example in diabetes mellitus

What is Leriche's syndrome?

Buttock claudication caused by atherosclerotic disease or saddle embolus at the aortic bifurcation

How might you investigate this patient?

ABPI/Exercise ABPI
Duplex ultrasound
Angiography/CTA/MRA

How could you manage a patient with peripheral vascular disease?

Conservative: risk factor modification, exercise, stop smoking
Medical: prophylactic antiplatelet and statin, control of diabetes if present
Surgical: endovascular, eg angioplasty +/- stent, or open procedure, such as thrombectomy, endarterectomy, patch angioplasty or bypass as appropriate

Examiner's Overall Assessment		
Pass	Fail	Borderline

TOP TIPS

 A full ABPI measurement may be too awkward or time-consuming during the examination, but you should certainly at least mention and describe it, as it is an essential part of a vascular exam.

2.3 Breast Examination

Common Scenarios
Breast exam is likely to be tested on a breast model for obvious reasons. Common cases you might encounter would include:

- Breast cancer
- Fibroadenoma
- Fibrocystic change

 Candidate Briefing

You are the SHO in breast clinic and have been asked to examine Mrs C who is a 47-year-old lady who has noticed a lump in her right breast. Please examine as you think necessary.

 Patient Briefing

You are Mrs C, a 47 year-old lady who presents with a lump in the upper outer quadrant of her right breast. This is non-tender. You have no other features of systemic disease and are well.

Examiner's Mark Scheme

Introduction	Mark (0-4)			
The candidate should: • Wash/gel hands, explain procedure, obtain consent • Ask for a chaperone and treat the patient with dignity at all times				

Exposure	Mark (0-4)			
• Expose the patient from the waist up and sit them on the edge of the bed. A sheet can be used to maintain dignity. • Ask patient to rest hands on thighs and relax arms and generally inspect breasts.				

OSCES

Inspection	Mark (0-4)			
• Look for asymmetry, skin changes such as peau d'orange, eczema, scars, obvious lumps or swellings and any nipple abnormalities such as inversion or discharge. • Ask patient to place her hands above her head and repeat the inspection • Repeat inspection again asking patient to put hands on hips and push inwards to tense pectoralis major. • Ask the patient to lie down with her arms by her sides and again repeat the general inspection.				

Palpation	Mark (0-4)			
• **Breasts**: Examine each breast individually starting with the normal side. Examine as a clock face with hand flat starting from the outside working inward toward the nipple. Patient has hand behind head of the breast that is being examined. • Palpate the nipple and the tissue deep to it. Mention discharge. • If lumps noted described in terms of site (as per clock face), size, shape, consistency, tethering to other structures.				
• **Axilla**: Examine both axillae for any enlarged lymph nodes - support the weight of that arm with your arm and examine with the other hand. Feel all three walls and the apex.				
• **Lymph nodes:** Palpate both supraclavicular fossa for any lymphadenopathy				

Closing	Mark (0-4)			
• Thanks patient • Maintains patient dignity				

OSCES

Presentation	Mark (0-4)			
• Summarise their findings • Offers an appropriate differential diagnosis and management plan • Suggests appropriate inital investigations such as arterial duplex				

Follow On Questions

What is meant by triple assessment?

Clinical examination, imaging and biopsy. Usually all performed in a one stop new breast referral clinic.

What forms of imaging do you know and when would they be used?

Ultrasound usually used in women of a younger age as they have denser breast tissue and better imaging.
Mammogram is first line in women over 50 years.
MRI is used in women with breast implants.

What is the UK's current breast screening programme?

Free service offered to women over 50 years up until the age of 70, every 3 years.

OSCES

Examiner's Overall Assessment		
Pass	Fail	Borderline

TOP TIPS

 Do not forget to palpate the nipple and the axillary tail of Spence, as cancers can be missed here and it shows you know how to do a thorough examination.

2.4 Cardiac Examination

Common Scenarios

This station could play out in a number of ways, either as an acute, ABCDE-type station, or in this case, more of a focused cardiac examination. Common cases you might see would include:

- Atrial Fibrillation *(AF)*
- Heart murmurs
- Evidence of previous cardiac surgery
- Myocardial infarction/acute heart failure *(simulated)*

 Candidate Briefing

Mr X is a 63-year-old gentleman who the ward nursing staff have asked you to see as he is complaining chest pain. Earlier today he underwent an elective open hernia repair.

He has hypertension and smokes 15 cigarettes a day.

He takes aspirin 75mg OD, Ramipril 5mg OD and simvastatin 40mg OD. On a brief history he says the pain is central and crushing in nature. He looks pale, anxious and sweaty.

Please examine the patient only, do not take any further detailed history.

 Patient Briefing

You are Mr/Mrs X, a 63 year-old patient who presents acutely unwell with chest pain following a hernia repair earlier on today. You have occasionally had similar discomfort after running for the bus but never this bad. You should appear in discomfort and slightly short of breath. You are anxious about what is happening.

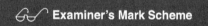 **Examiner's Mark Scheme**

Introduction	Mark (0-4)			
The candidate should: • Wash/gel hands, explain procedure, obtain consent • Ask for a chaperone and treat the patient with dignity at all times				

OSCES

Inspection	Mark (0-4)			
• Comment on general condition of the patient from the end of the bed • Position patient at 45 degrees with chest exposed. • Comment on other bedside features, such as monitoring leads etc				
• **Peripheral:** Inspects hands, face and lower limbs for peripheral stigmata of cardiovascular disease e.g. clubbing, central cyanosis, oedema and vein harvesting scars.				
• **Chest:** Inspects for scars and deformity				

Palpation	Mark (0-4)			
• **Peripheral:** Asks for or take patient's pulse, requests blood pressure and 3 lead ECG monitoring assesses JVP • Compares peripheral pulses				
• **Chest:** Palpates carotid pulse, feels for apex beat and heaves				

Auscultation	Mark (0-4)			
• Listen to heart sounds in all four regions with pulse to define diastolic, pan-systolic and ejection systolic murmurs.				
• **Chest:** Palpates carotid pulse, feels for apex beat and heaves • Perform specific manoeuvres to elicit murmurs				

Closing	Mark (0-4)			
• Thanks patient • Maintains patient dignity				

Presentation	Mark (0-4)			
• Summarise their findings • Offers an appropriate differential diagnosis and management plan • Suggests appropriate inital investigations such as an ECG, CXR, ECHO etc.				

OSCES

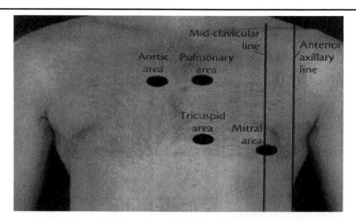

Follow On Questions

You requested an ECG. The most obvious abnormality is ST eleva-tion in II, III and aVF. There is Q-wave formation in III and aVF and reciprocal ST depression and T wave inversion in aVL. What does this suggest?

This pattern suggests an inferior myocardial infarction.

What would be your management of this patient?

ABCD. GTN and morphine, oxygen. Manage in line with local cardiac chest pain protocol. An urgent serum troponin should be sent- if raised, or if the ECG demonstrates ischaemic changes, he needs full anticoagulation with aspirin or clopidogrel, and low molecular weight heparin. As he is post-operative, this requires discussion with the vascular consultant as to risk of bleeding versus benefit of anti-coagulation for myocardial infarction. Also will require discussion with on call cardiologist as primary coronary intervention may be an option.

You heard a mitral regurgitation murmur that you cannot see has been noted before, what is a sensible first line investigation to request?

Echocardiography

Examiner's Overall Assessment		
Pass	Fail	Borderline

TOP TIPS

 This station could play out in a number of ways, either as an acute, ABCDE-type station, or in this case, more of a focused cardiac examination. it might be worth using the examiner to direct you, perhaps by starting with a brief ABC assessment and then asking 'would you like me to proceed to more detailed cardiovascular examination?'

2.5   Cerebellar Examination

Common Scenarios

Cerebellar lesions are unusual in the examination. Causes of headaches and dizziness are legion, but the vignette directs you a cerebellar examination. These include:

- Tumours
- Strokes
- Neurodegenerative disorders
- Head trauma

 Candidate Briefing

Mr Bristol is an 81 year old gentleman who presents with headaches and dizziness. Please perform a cerebellar examination.

 Patient Briefing

You are Mr/Mrs Bristol, you are an 81 year-old who has had headaches for a few months, but they have been much worse more recently and now you also feel dizzy. You feel otherwise well in yourself and cannot remember any particular event that seemed to set all this off. You are otherwise relaxed and happy to let the doctor examine you and tell you what is going on. When examined, you should have some dysdiadochokinesia (difficult doing repeated alternating movements), intention tremor (shaking when you try and complete a movement with your hands) and past pointing.

⌣⌢ Examiner's Mark Scheme

Introduction	Mark (0-4)			
• Wash/gel hands, explain procedure, obtain consent • Ask for a chaperone and treat the patient with dignity at all times • Stop the candidate if they start doing a general neurological examination initially. If there is time at the end of the cerebellar examination the candidate can do a general neurological examination.				

Inspection	Mark (0-4)			
• Perform a general inspection, commenting on obvious signs of neurological dysfunction • Comment on other bedside features				

Examination	Mark (0-4)			
• **D**: Examine for dysdiadochokinesia. Ask patient to place back of their hand onto their other palm and then turn the top hand over, repeat process, increasing speed and repeat to examine the other side. Positive sign is inability to perform rapid alternating movements				
• **A**: Examine for ataxia. Ask the patient to walk in front of you. Ataxia is demonstrated through a broad based gait with difficulty in turning				
• **N**: Examine for nystagmus. Oscillating movement of the eyes. Check eye movements, particularly apparent at extremes of gaze				
• **I**: Examine for intention tremor. Ask patient to point from their nose to the candidate's finger. Ensure finger is at arms length. Finger should be moved to different positions. As the patient approaches the candidate's finger a tremor may be noticed.				
• **S**: Examine for slurred speech/dysarthria. May be noticed in general conversation. Asks the patient to say different phrases, for example, "baby hippopotamus"; "British constitution".				
• **H**: Examine for hypotonia. Candidate examines upper and lower limb tone by rolling patients lower legs and moving patient's arms.				
• **P**: Examine for past pointing. Assessed when looking for intention tremor. The patient will point past the candidate's fingertip if present.				

OSCES

Closing	Mark (0-4)			
• Thanks patient • Maintains patient dignity				

Presentation	Mark (0-4)			
• Summarise their findings • Offers an appropriate differential diagnosis and management plan • Suggests appropriate inital investigations such as bloods, MRI head				

Follow On Questions

If this patient had positive signs what follow-up investigations would you order?

Basic bloods, including full blood count and calcium. Plain chest radiography. A CT head is important, but an MRI will provide much better imaging of the posterior fossa.

When would you organise a head CT rather than an MRI?

Head CT- quick, good for bleeds (acute pathology), contrast versus non-contrast. MRI- better definition of structural layers, better for tumours, A-V malformations however not as readily available and patients will wait longer.

What is the most common tumour affecting the cerebellum?

Metastases, astrocytoma in adults, medulloblastoma in children.

Examiner's Overall Assessment		
Pass	Fail	Borderline

TOP TIPS

 The DANISH mnemonic is useful here to remember the components of a cerebellar examination, which can be confusing. Avoid the stumbling block of trying to fit everything in by stating to the examiner *"I am going to examine specifically for posterior fossa lesions – to complete my examination I would do a full neurological examination and history"*.

OSCES

2.6 | Cranial Nerve Examination

Common Scenarios

This could be a normal examination or present with a number of features, likely simulated given the nature of the station. These may include:

- Haemotympanum or other evidence of base of skull fracture
- Cranial nerve lesion – particularly 3rd or 6th nerve palsy

 Candidate Briefing

You are the surgical SHO on-call. Mr X, a 24-year-old, hit his head during a game of rugby and has been brought to A&E by paramedics. They tell you he was unconscious for approximately 30 seconds afterwards, then recovering spontaneously and has since been alert and orientated. He complains of a headache. Please perform a cranial nerve examination.

😐 **Patient Briefing**

You are Mr X, a 24 year-old fit and well man. You hit your head playing rugby and think you were knocked out, but now you feel ok, apart from a banging headache. If asked, you should also say that you feel your hearing in your left ear is reduced. Your vision is fine and you have no other abnormal findings on examination.

 Examiner's Mark Scheme

Introduction	Mark (0-4)			
• Wash/gel hands, explain procedure, obtain consent • Ask for a chaperone and treat the patient with dignity at all times				

Inspection	Mark (0-4)			
• A thorough inspection of the patient's face and scalp, commenting on important negatives such as absence of lacerations, bruising (particularly panda eyes/Battle's sign) and neurological stigmata e.g. Pupil inequality.				

• May gain an additional mark for palpating the patient's face for steps and crepitus,and examining teeth opposition				

Examination	Mark (0-4)			
• **CN1:** Mentions would test smell if any concerns.				
• **CN2**: Tests light and accommodation reflexes, fields, acuity, mentions fundoscopy (not necessary to perform so instruct the candidate to move on if begins to examine fundi.				
• **CN3, 4, 6**: Examines eye movements.				
• **CN5:** Tests sensation on forehead, cheeks, mandible. Palpates contracted Masseter and Temporalis muscles.				
• **CN7**: Tests motor function of 5 divisions of facial nerve. May mention taste to anterior 2/3 of tongue.				
• **CN8**: Should examine ears for haemotympanum (or comment on this if Otoscope unavailable). Crude test of hearing deficit. Should do Rinne and Weber tests if tuning fork available.				
• **CN9**: Should ask patient to swallow and to say Ahh, examining for uvula deviation. Mention gag reflex.				
• **CN10:** Should ask patient to cough. May mention speech difficulties. Also tested by gag reflex.				
• **CN11:** Shrug shoulders (Trapezius), turn head to left and right (SCM).				
• **CN12:** Tongue protusion and deviation.				

Closing	Mark (0-4)		
• Thanks patient • Maintains patient dignity			

Presentation	Mark (0-4)		
• Summarise their findings • Offers an appropriate differential diagnosis and management plan • Suggests appropriate inital investigations such as bloods, MRI head			

Follow On Questions

Describe the components of the Glasgow Coma Scale

• **Motor**: obeys commands, localizes pain, withdraws, abnormal flexion, abnormal extension, no movement
• **Voice**: normal speech, confused speech, inappropriate words, occasional groans, no speech
• **Eyes**: open spontaneously, to voice, to pain, closed

What are the classic CT features of extradural and subdural haematomas?

• Extradural are typically lenticuloform or ellipse-shaped (due to the spread of blood being limited by attachments of the dura to the skull, where as subdurals are cresenteric and spread without restriction over the surface of the brain.

How may traumatic brain injury be classified, using the GCS scale?

• Mild or minor - 13-15
• Moderate – 9-12
• Severe – 3-8
• Vegetative – 3

Examiner's Overall Assessment		
Pass	Fail	Borderline

TOP TIPS

 Don't miss any clues as to what examination the examiners want you to perform – for example, there may be an otoscope or ophthalmoscope on the table in the station. This is there for a reason – make sure you use it in your examination!

OSCES

2.7 | Hand Examination

Common Scenarios

Hand conditions can lead to excellent signs for the purposes of examination. Common cases may include:

- Rheumatoid arthritis
- Psoriasis/psoriatic arthritis
- Scleroderma
- Osteoarthritis
- Traumatic injury/amputation

 Candidate Briefing

Mr/Mrs Y is a 45 year-old lady whom has been referred by her GP complaining of gradually worsening pain and swelling affecting her hands. She works as a secretary and has found her work has been affected. Please examine her as you see fit, then answer the examiner's questions.

 Patient Briefing

You are Mr/Mrs Y. a 45 year-old secretary who presents with painful, swollen hands. On examination they should be globally stiff and tender, particularly at the metacarpo-phalangeal joints. Dexterity should be reasonable but you should complain that it is not as good as it used to be, and typing has become more difficult.

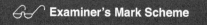 **Examiner's Mark Scheme**

Introduction	Mark (0-4)			
• Wash/gel hands, explain procedure, obtain consent • Ask for a chaperone and treat the patient with dignity at all times				

Inspection	Mark (0-4)			
• Thoroughly inspect the patient's hands; commenting on swelling, erythema, classic deformities (z-thumb, swan neck, boutonniere), muscle wasting, scars and nail signs.				
• Should look at elbows for plaques and general patient inspection also				
• May perform some screening tests, such as asking patient to undo a button, pick up a coin or similar				

Palpation	Mark (0-4)			
• **Temperature**: warm, swollen joints are indicative of active disease.				
• **Wrist Joint Margins**: palpate the ulna head, radial styloid and carpal bones. Pain over the anatomical snuff box may indicate a scaphoid fracture. Tenderness over the ulna head is found in extensor carpi ulnaris tendinitis and pain over the radial styloid may indicate de Quervain's tenosynovitis.				
• **Carpal Joint Margins**: look at the patient's face to see if this is tender. Feel whether the joint is soft (rheumatoid) or hard (osteoarthritis or gouty tophi). Squeeze the MCP joints noting whether this is painful (active disease). Palpate the individual joints.				

Movement	Mark (0-4)			
Active then passive movement of the wrist then carpal joints (comparing both hands):				
Wrist Flexion (0-80°): put your hands together in a prayer sign				
Wrist Extension (0-70°): put the back your hands together in a reverse prayer sign				

Movement	Mark (0-4)			
Ulna (0-40°): bend the wrist so that the little finger nears the ulnar				
Radial Deviation (0-20°): bend the wrist so the thumb nears the radius				
Finger Flexion/Extension (0-90°): make a fist and straighten the fingers out				
Finger abduction: spread your fingers out, testing the dorsal interossei supplied by the ulnar nerve				

Special Tests	Mark (0-4)			
Carpal tunnel syndrome • Tinnel's Sign: Tap on their wrist repeatedly to reveal tingling in the median nerve distribution • Phalen's Sign: Hold hands in forced flexion (reverse prayer sign), this maneuver causes median nerve compression eliciting carpal tunnel symptoms.				
Ulnar Nerve Function • Froment's Sign: Ask patient to hold a piece of paper between thumb and finger, tests adductor pollicis. Those with ulnar nerve palsy find it difficult to effectively grip the paper.				
De Quervain's Tenosynovitis • Finkelstein's Test: Ask the patient to flex the thumb then deviate the wrist to the ulnar side. Pain on this movement indicates De Quervain's Tenosynovitis.				

Neurological • Tone: patient flexes/extends fingers in a wave. Ask them to open and close their hands very quickly (slow in myotonica dystrophica)				

- Power:
  Median: patient gives 'thumbs up'. Patient makes 'ok sign' for anterior interosseous branch.
  Ulnar: patient abducts all fingers
  Radial: patient extends wrist/metacarpals
- Sensation: check pinprick and light touch just in one area for each nerve
  Median: lateral thumb
  Ulnar: medial little finger
  Radial: anatomical snuffbox

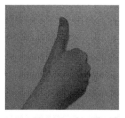

Median

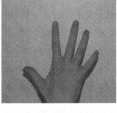

Ulna nerve

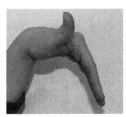

Radial nerve

OSCES

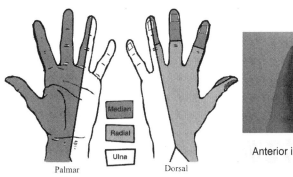

Palmar   Dorsal

Median
Radial
Ulna

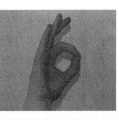

Anterior interosseous

Presentation	Mark (0-4)			
• Summarise their findings • Offers an appropriate differential diagnosis and management plan • Offers to examine the joint above and request radiographs				

Follow On Questions

Describe the characteristic deformities seen in rheumatoid arthritis

- Swan neck – hyperextension at PIPJ, flexion at DIPJ
- Bouttoniere – flexion at PIPJ, hyperextension at DIPJ
- Z-Thumb – flexion at MCPJ, extension at IPJ
- Radial deviation at wrist joint
- Ulnar deviation and subluxation at MCPJs

What are the classic x-ray features of rheumatoid arthritis?

- Joint space narrowing
- Ill-defined bony erosions
- Juxta-articular osteopaenia
- Soft tissue swelling

How may RA be managed?

- Conservative: splinting, activity modification, physiotherapy
- Medical: NSAIDs, DMARDs, Biological agents
- Surgery: arthroscopic washout/synovectomy, arthroplasty

Examiner's Overall Assessment		
Pass	Fail	Borderline

TOP TIPS

 The optimal set-up for this examination is with the patient sat and the examining doctor sat opposite them. The patient should rest their arms on a pillow or low table so that they are relaxed and comfortable. Taking the time to get this setup shows concern for the patient and permits a relaxed and effective inspection and examination.

2.8 Hernia Examination

Common Scenarios

Hernias are often seen in the exam and may incude:

- Inguinal *(direct/indirect)*
- Epigastric
- Incisional
- Paraumbilical
- Femoral
- Spigelian *(rare)*

 Candidate Briefing

You are a surgical SHO in the general surgical clinic. Mr P is a 45-year-old who noticed a lump in his right groin 6 months ago, now getting larger and occasionally sore. Please examine the patient as you feel appropriate and present your findings to the examiner.

OSCES

 Patient Briefing

You are Mr P, a 45 year-old fit and well man who noticed a lump in his right groin several months ago. It is painful and you notice it particularly when coughing/sneezing. It comes out but you are able to push it back. On examination you are tender in the right inguinal region but say the lump is reduced currently.

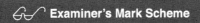 **Examiner's Mark Scheme**

Introduction	Mark (0-4)			
• Wash/gel hands, explain procedure, obtain consent • Ask for a chaperone and treat the patient with dignity at all times				

Inspection	Mark (0-4)			
• Mention full exposure 'nipple to knee' but indicate they can continue fully clothed/partially exposed				
• Perform general inspection, commenting on the patient's overall appearance				
• Comment on the hernia itself, including position, scrotal extension, skin changes, scars				

Palpation	Mark (0-4)			
Palpate the hernia and assess the following:				
• Able to get above - unlikely to be a hernia				
• Extension into scrotum - likely indirect				
• Cough impulse				
• Reducible or irreducible (signaling impending or current incarceration)				
• Tenderness (another sign of impending incarceration/strangulation)				
• Differentiation between indirect & direct including occlusion of deep inguinal ring (at the mid-point of the inguinal ligament) & coughing- indirect hernias remain reduced, direct reappear.				

Auscultation	Mark (0-4)			
• Listen for bowel sounds				

Closing	Mark (0-4)			
• Thanks patient • Maintains patient dignity				

Presentation	Mark (0-4)			
• Summarise their findings • Offers an appropriate differential diagnosis and management plan • Offers to examine the abdomen and external genitalia				

Follow On Questions

What are the major complications of inguinal herniae?

Bowel obstruction & strangulation

Please define bowel strangulation

Strangulation is constriction of bowel preventing venous return causing venous congestion, arterial occlusion and ischaemia. This may lead to perforation. This is a surgical emergency and requires urgent repair.

Describe the borders of the inguinal canal

• The inguinal ligament (and the lacunar ligament medially) forms the floor. The roof is the arching fibres of the transversus abdominis and internal oblique.
• The anterior wall is the external oblique aponeurosis. The posterior border is formed by the transversalis fascia laterally and the conjoint tendon along its medial one third.
• At the lateral end of the canal is the deep inguinal ring at the mid-point of the inguinal ligament (halfway between the ASIS and pubic tubercle).
• The superficial inguinal ring lies medially, it is just superior and medial to the pubic tubercle.

List the contents of the inguinal canal

The inguinal canal contains the spermatic cord in males and the round ligament in females. It also contains the ilioinguinal nerve in both.

Spermatic cord contents are as follows:
• **3 arteries:** testicular artery (branch of aorta), artery of the vas, cremasteric artery (branch of inferior epigastric)
• **3 nerves**: genital branch of the genitofemoral nerve (L1/2), sympathetics, ilioinguinal nerve (L1, not technically in the cord)
• **3 fascial layers**: external spermatic (from external oblique), cremasteric (from internal oblique), internal spermatic (from transversalis fascia)
• **3 others**: vas deferens, pampiniform plexus, lymphatic vessels

Examiner's Overall Assessment		
Pass	Fail	Borderline

TOP TIPS

 Don't forget to consider other differentials for a groin lump, eg saphena varix, lymphadenopathy, femoral artery aneurysm etc.

2.9 Hip Joint Examination

Common Scenarios
Certainly a popular station in the examine. You would be likely to see:
- Osteoarthritis
- Post-traumatic arthritis
- Rheumatoid arthritis

 Candidate Briefing

Mr/Mrs X is a 72 year old who has presented complaining of right hip pain. He/she has a history of hypertension, which is well controlled, and type 2 diabetes for which he/she takes metformin. He/she has been managing the pain with simple analgesia to date but recently has been struggling more and is finding it affects his/her activities of daily life. Please examine his/her hip, present your findings and then answer any questions from the examiner.

 Patient Briefing

You are Mr/Mrs X, a 72 year-old with a painful right hip. On examination you should have an antalgic gait but normal trendelenburg test. Your hip should be stiff and painful when moved, particularly in internal rotation.

OSCES

Examiner's Mark Scheme

Introduction	Mark (0-4)			
• Wash/gel hands, explain procedure, obtain consent • Ask for a chaperone and treat the patient with dignity at all times				

Inspection	Mark (0-4)			
Asking the patient to walk a short distance is a good screening test and allows you to combine 'looking' at the hip and leg, analysing gait and looking for any gross deformity.				

Gait				
• Antalgic: shorter steps due to pain, the commonest cause is OA. • Scissor: legs move with a rigid outward swing resembling a pair of scissors . Due to hypertonic legs, associated with UMN lesion particularly cerebral palsy • Trendelenburg: weakness of abductor muscles. The pelvis sags on the opposite side of the superior gluteal nerve lesion • Ataxic: unsteady, broad-based gait associated with cerebellar dysfunction. • High Stepping/Foot drop: due to loss of dorsiflexion secondary to peroneal nerve injury. The patient is unable to dorsiflex and compensates with a high step prior to landing the foot.				
• Check the front and back then position them on the examination couch **Skin**: Scars (check buttocks), swelling, venous/arterial disease. **Muscle**: Wasting of the quads/glutei/hamstrings **Bone & Joint:** Length, deformities (e.g. leg shortened or externally rotated)				

Palpation	Mark (0-4)		
Measure Position the pelvis so ASIS at same level • True length: Distance from medial malleolus to ASIS each side • Apparent length: Distance from medial malleolus to bottom of sternum			
Palpate for bony prominences. Greater Trochanter, ASIS, iliac crests, pubic rami. The hip is deep so tenderness is unlikely			

Movement	Mark (0-4)		
Active Movements: The patient moves Passive Movements: The doctor moves Compare each side			
• **Flexion (0-120°):** bring your knee up to your stomach			

OSCES

• **Extension (0-10°)**: best done with the patient standing or lying prone, move leg backwards.				
• **Abduction (0-45°)**: with a straight leg move the leg outwards				
• **Adduction (0-30°):** with a straight leg move the leg across to the opposite side				
• **External Rotation (0-45°):** rotate thigh outwards				
• **Internal Rotation (0-30°):** rotate thigh inwards, do this with the knee and hip flexed				

Special Tests	Mark (0-4)			
Although 'Special Tests' are often left till the end of the examination, while you have the patient standing, now is a good time to perform Trendelenberg's Test to assess abductor function. **Trendelenburg's Test** Stand in front of the patient facing them and take their hands in yours. Ask the patient to stand on one leg. Normally the pelvis tilts up on unsupported side (abductors on weight bearing side). A positive Trendelenburg is when the unsupported side droops, indicating pathology on the leg on which they are standing. A mnemonic is: "sound side sags", indicating the normal leg which is in the air sags. Causes: weakness of the abductors, dislocation/fractures, pain, fixed flexion deformity.				
Thomas' Test (fixed flexion deformity) Fully flex both legs to obliterate lumbar lordosis (can place one hand under back to confirm). Hold one leg fully flexed and straighten the other. The patient should be able to lie the other leg fully on to the bed, any angle left is the degree of fixed flexion. Repeat on other side.				

Presentation	Mark (0-4)		
• Summarise their findings • Offers an appropriate differential diagnosis and management plan • Offers to examine the joint above and below and request radiographs			

Follow On Questions

What do you think the diagnosis is?

Osteoarthritis: conceivably primary, or secondary (post-traumatic). Differentials include trochanteric bursitis, femoroacetabular impingement, obturator hernia, stress fracture, bony malignancy (primary or secondary)

What investigations could you organise to demonstrate this?

X-rays, CT, MRI, diagnostic hip injection

What are the characteristic features of osteoarthritis on plain radiographs?

Joint space narrowing, subchondral sclerosis, subchondral cyst formation and osteophytosis

How would you manage this condition?

Conservative: physio/OT, activity modification, heat
Medical: paracetamol, NSAIDs, opiates – WHO ladder, steroid injection
Surgical: arthroplasty

Examiner's Overall Assessment		
Pass	Fail	Borderline

TOP TIPS

A good screening test for gross hip irritability is internal/external rotation with the leg extended in the supine position

2.10 Neck Lump Examination

Common Scenarios

There are many causes for neck lumps, but lymphadenopathy and subcutaneous lesions such as lipomas are most likely to be seen in the exam.

 Candidate Briefing

Mr X is a 27 year-old man who has presented complaining of a lump in his neck. Please examine him as you see fit, then answer the examiner's questions.

 Patient Briefing

You are Mr/Mrs X, a 27 year-old patient with a lump in the left side of your neck. You're not sure how long it has been there, but you are quite anxious about it as you are worried it might be a cancer. It is non-tender and you have no other abnormal findings.

OSCES

Examiner's Mark Scheme

Introduction	Mark (0-4)			
• Wash/gel hands, explain procedure, obtain consent • Ask for a chaperone and treat the patient with dignity at all times				

Inspection	Mark (0-4)			
• Inspect whole patient, commenting on appearance and stigmata of thyroid or haematological disease, including facial stigmata				

Inspection	Mark (0-4)			
• Perform thorough inspection of the neck, commenting on obvious masses, skin changes, scars and other abnormalities				
• Asks patient to sip water provided and inspects neck with water held and then on swallowing				

Palpation	Mark (0-4)			
• Systematic palpation of mass and whole of neck, including various lymph node regions and thyroid				
• Ask patient to protrude their tongue or swallow, and assess movement of any neck mass				
• Ask to palpate structures in the mouth – tell them this isn't necessary but award a point if mentioned				
• Assess fluctuance, pulsatility and transilluminability				

Closing	Mark (0-4)			
• Thanks patient • Maintains patient dignity				

Presentation	Mark (0-4)			
• Summarise their findings • Offers an appropriate differential diagnosis and management plan • Offers to examine the joint above and below and request radiographs				
• Presentation should comment on any mass/es, including size, shape, surface, surroundings, consistency/fluctuance, fixity/tethering, location, temperature, pulsatility, transillumination				

Follow On Questions

What are your differentials?

Lymph node, parotid mass, sebaceous cyst, lipoma, abscess, carotid body tumour, branchial cyst

What investigations would you wish to perform?

Routine bloods, ultrasound, fine needle aspiration, excision biopsy, CT/MRI

What is a cystic hygroma?

This is a congenital malformation of the lymphatics, causing a unilateral multi-loculated cystic lesion found potentially anywhere but usually in the posterior triangle of the neck or the armpits.

On the approach to the submandibular gland, where should your incision be, and why?

This should be at least 2 fingerbreadths below the mandible, to avoid damaging the mandibular nerve.

Describe the borders of the triangles of the neck

•The anterior triangle is bordered by the midline medially, the SCM posterolaterally and the body of the mandible superiorly. Within the anterior triangle are 4 subdivisions: Muscular (midline, SCM, omohyoid); Carotid (SCM, omohyoid, posterior digastric); Submandibular (mandible, anterior and posterior bellies of digastric); Submental (midline, anterior digastric, hyoid)
• The posterior triangle is bordered by the SCM anteriorly, the clavicle inferiorly and the edge of trapezius posteriorly. It has 2 subdivisions: Occipital (SCM, trapezius, omohyoid) and Subclavian (omohyoid, clavicle, SCM)

Describe the Memorial Sloan Kettering Cancer Centre boundaries of the neck.

The midline is the central dividing line.
• **Level I:** submental and submandibular. Along the body of the mandible to the angle, then inferomedially to the hyoid bone and then superomedially back to the mandible.
• **Level II**: upper sternomastoid. The upper third of the sternomastoid above the level of the hyoid bone.
• **Level III:** middle sternomastoid. The middle third of the sternomastoid between the level of the hyoid bone and the level of the cricoid cartilage.
• **Level IV**: lower sternomastoid. The lower third of the sternomastoid beneath the level of the cricoid cartilage.
• **Level V:** posterior triangle. The triangle formed by the posterior border of sternomastoid, anterior border of trapezius and superior border of the clavicle.
• **Level VI:** anterior compartment. The anterior part of the neck along the hyoid bone to its lateral tip then inferiorly along the anterior border of sternomastoid.

Examiner's Overall Assessment		
Pass	Fail	Borderline

TOP TIPS

 Like the wound station, make a point of vocalising your examination to the examiner, either during or after, to make it obvious that you have examined thoroughly for all the characteristics listed above. Complete your examination by saying you would palpate other regions for lymphadenopathy, such as the axillae and groins.

OSCES

2.11 Knee Joint Examination

Common Scenarios

Another common station in the exam. You may see:

- Osteoarthritis and associated deformities
- Rheumatoid arthritis
- Post-traumatic arthritis
- Ligamentous laxity
- Post-surgical findings

Candidate Briefing

Mr/Mrs X is a 57 year old who has presented complaining of knee pain. He/she has a history of asthma, which is well controlled. He/she has been managing the pain with simple analgesia to date but recently has been struggling more and is finding it affects his/her work. Please examine his/her knees, present your findings and then answer any questions from the examiner

Patient Briefing

You are Mr/Mrs X, a 57 year-old patient with a painful right knee. You should walk with a limp and, on examination, have reduced flexion and joint line tenderness.

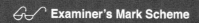

Examiner's Mark Scheme

Introduction	Mark (0-4)			
• Wash/gel hands, explain procedure, obtain consent • Ask for a chaperone and treat the patient with dignity at all times				
• Checks that patient isn't in pain				

Inspection	Mark (0-4)			
Asking the patient to walk a short distance is a good screening test and allows gross assessment of mobility				
Inspect whilst standing • Skin: Scars, swelling, erythema • Muscle: Quadriceps wasting, effusions • Bone & Joint: Valgus/varus deformity. Valgus = knees come together, varus = bow-legged				

Palpation	Mark (0-4)			
• Sits the patient on the examination couch and look at their flexed knee • Palpates the joint line				
• With the patient sitting you may wish to test patella tracking Place your thumb and middle finger either side of the patella and use your index finger to feel the top of the patella Ask the patient to extend their knee from a flexed position				
With the patient lying supine compare sides. • Temperature: compare sides with the back of your hand				
• Stroke test for effusions: empty the medial compartment with your hand by massaging fluid up and into the lateral side. Then apply pressure over lateral side whilst holding your other hand above the patella. Watch the medial gutter whilst doing this: it will balloon if there is an effusion.				
• Palpate Joint Margin: Bend knee to 90 degrees with foot on bed. Palpate joint line for tenderness (meniscal pathology), and the medial/lateral collaterals				
• Examine popliteal fossa for cysts, aneurysm				

Movement	Mark (0-4)			
Active then passive movements. For passive movements keep one hand over the knee for crepitus.				
• **Flexion (0-130°):** bend their leg whilst putting a hand on their knee and feeling for crepitus. Their heel should be able to touch their buttocks				
• **Extension (0-15°):** Lift the patients leg in the air with your hand on their ankle (ask the patient to let you take their weight). If the leg extends fully then there is no fixed flexion				

Special Tests	Mark (0-4)			
• **Collateral ligaments**: flex knee to 20 degrees and apply varus/valgus stress				
• **Anterior/posterior draw test:** With the knee at 90 degrees, look from the side for sag of tibia in relation to femur (tear of posterior cruciate). Now anchor the foot by sitting on the end of the toes (be very careful not to hurt the patient). Grab the leg below the knee with both hands and push it back (posterior draw for posterior cruciate tear) and pull forward (anterior draw test for anterior cruciate tear).				
• **Lachman's Test** for anterior cruciate injury: bend the patient's leg to 30 degrees and grasp above the knee with one hand and below with the other. Apply slow pressure to the back of the proximal tibia (below the knee), increased laxness indicates injury.				
• **McMurray's test** for meniscal tears: McMurray's test is performed with the patient lying flat (non-weight bearing). Bend the knee and place one hand on the lateral side to stabilize the joint and provide a valgus stress. The other hand rotates the leg externally while extending the knee. A click is felt over the meniscus tear as the knee is brought from full flexion to 90 degrees of flexion.				

OSCES

Presentation	Mark (0-4)			
• Summarise their findings • Offers an appropriate differential diagnosis and management plan • Offers to examine the joint above and below and request radiographs				

Follow On Questions

What do you think the diagnosis is?

Osteoarthritis.
Differentials include ligamentous injury, rheumatological disease eg gout, rheumatoid arthritis etc, bony tumour (primary or secondary).

What investigations could you organise to demonstrate this?

X-rays, MRI, possibly diagnostic arthroscopy

How would you manage this condition?

Conservative: physio/OT, activity modification, heat
Medical: paracetamol, NSAIDs, opiates – WHO ladder, steroid injection
Surgical: arthroplasty

What is the most common deformity seen with osteoarthritis of the knee?

Varus deformity

Examiner's Overall Assessment		
Pass	Fail	Borderline

TOP TIPS

Remember to compare sides. Some patients may have slight hypermobility or lax ACLs.

OSCES

2.12 Wound Management

Common Scenarios

The usual format in the exam is to have an actor with a simulated "wound" – usually a big cut in a piece of foam, or possible a bit of meat, similar to the basic surgical skills courses.

 Candidate Briefing

You are the orthopaedic SHO on call and are asked to see Mr B in the ED department. He is a 26 year old gentleman who earlier whilst intoxicated got into an altercation and punched his right arm through a glass window. Please assess and treat the wound as appropriate.

This station is a test of practical skill. You may like to practice with a suturing kit to become familiar with the equipment. Please close the wound using the equipment provided.

 Patient Briefing

You are Mr/Mrs B, a 26-year-old who got drunk and upset earlier and punched a window, cutting your arm. You are calm and cooperative now and generally should not interfere with the candidate's examination, other than to ask whether you will have a scar and whether you have any tendon damage.

Examiner's Mark Scheme

Introduction	Mark (0-4)			
• Wash/gel hands, explain procedure, obtain consent				
• Confirms area of injury and plan. Checks allergies and patient info				

Skin Preparation	Mark (0-4)			
• Cleans skin with appropriate chlorhexadine solution				

Anaesthetic	Mark (0-4)			
• Anaesthetise with local anaesthestic using field block				

Suture Selection	Mark (0-4)			
• Choose a non-absorbable suture such as a 3-0/ 4-0 prolene on a cutting needle				

Needle Handling	Mark (0-4)			
• Uses needle holders to handle needle at all times				

Suturing	Mark (0-4)			
• Use interrupted sutures				
• Appropriate distnace between sutures				
• Securely ties each suture				
• Cuts sutures to appropriate length				

Sharps Disposal	Mark (0-4)			
• Safely disposes sharps into provided sharps bin				

Follow On Questions

How would you initially assess the wound?

- Site of wound
- Size of wound
- Level of contamination
- Underlying structural damage
- Neurovascular status
- Patient's pain level

What investigations would you order?

X-ray for foreign bodies or underlying fracture

If there was a fracture how would it change your management?

If a fracture is present it needs to be treated as an open fracture and the patient admitted for IV antibiotics, washout and debridement in theatre

There is no fracture and you decide to close his arm laceration in ED. Please describe how you would go about this?

- Introduce self and consent
- Anaesthetise wound with local anaesthetic
- Remove any large debris
- Washout the wound with 1L saline until visibly clean
- Assess for the base of the wound and rule out any other structural damage
- Suture the wound together
- Check tetanus status

When would you decide to close the wound in theatre as oppose to in ED?

If too large to anaesthetise locally, grossly contaminated, patient uncooperative, other structures damaged requiring repair (ie tendons and nerves), open joints

What type of local anaesthetic would you use and what are maximum doses?

Lignocaine with adrenaline, No adrenaline if end structure/digit
Lignocaine 3mg/kg, 7mg/kg if adrenaline
Bupivacaine 2mg/kg

What are the signs of LA toxicity?

Periorbital tingling, severe agitation, loss of consciousness, tonic-clonic seizure

What follow-up information would you give him before discharge?

- Keep wound clean and dry
- See GP in 7 – 10 days for removal of sutures
- Advise on signs of a wound infection

Examiner's Overall Assessment		
Pass	Fail	Borderline

TOP TIPS

 Talk through what you are doing as you are doing it, to ensure the examiner is able to tick all the boxes and give you full marks. You can either do this as you do your examination, or just state everything you have looked for having done your inspection.

2.13 Respiratory Examination

Common Scenarios
This is another case that requires some acutely ill patient assessment, ie an ABCDE approach. It is likely to be simulated for obvious reasons. Non-acute diagnoses might include COPD or fibrosing alveolitis.

 Candidate Briefing

Mrs C is a 52-year-old patient who the ward nurse has asked you to see as she is complaining of difficulty breathing. She is due to have an emergency cholecystectomy tomorrow. She has a background of COPD and smokes 15 cigarettes a day. She uses several regular inhalers but no home oxygen. On a brief history she says she has missed several regular inhalers & has a tight chest. She cannot complete full sentences, is pale, anxious and wheezy.
Please examine the patient only, do not take any further detailed history.

 Patient Briefing

You are Mrs C, a 52 year-old lady who is acutely short of breath. You are awaiting an emergency operation to take out your gallbladder tomorrow. You should be anxious, short of breath and complain that your chest feels very tight. You should be unable to talk in full sentences and wheezy.

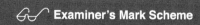 **Examiner's Mark Scheme**

Introduction	Mark (0-4)			
• Wash/gel hands, explain procedure, obtain consent				
• Checks patient is comfortable and not in pain				

OSCES

Inspection	Mark (0-4)			
• Comment on general condition of the patient from the end of the bed • Looks around bed for: medication, oxygen, insulin, chest leads, walking aids, medical-alert bracelet. • Does the patient look: well, breathless, well nourished. Any recognisable syndrome, how is the patient's complexion?				
Peripheral • Inspect dorsal and palmar aspects of hand-snoting colour, skin texture, deformities and feel for temperature or sweating. Look for tar-staining, finger clubbing • Nails: koilonychias (spoon-shaped nail in iron deficiency), onycholysis (destruction), Beau's lines (chronic disease), Mee's lines (renal failure), Muehrcke's lines (hypoalbu-minaemia), pitting (psoriasis/alopecia) and capillary nailbed pulsation (Quinke's sign of aortic regurge). • Wrists: for tenderness (hypertrophic pulmo-nary osteoarthropathy – lung ca), asterixis (CO_2 retention flap, liver failure). Test for CO_2 retention flap. 'Can you stretch out your arms and cock your wrists.' • Mouth: Looking for central cyanosis				
Chest • Assess praecordium for scars (look in apex) and ask patient to identify, implantable devices, colour, surface vessels, muscular deformity, breathing.				

Palpation	Mark (0-4)			
• Chest expansion (both hands, thumbs meet in midline below nipples – reduced expansion implies pathology on that side)				

Percussion	Mark (0-4)			
• Percuss for resonant (normal), hyper-resonant (pneumothorax), dull (consolidation) or stony dull (pleural effusion) note.				

Auscultation	Mark (0-4)			
• Listen to lung fields, listen with diaphragm over same areas percussed Breathe sounds: normally vesicular. Bronchial breathing indicates consolidation. Reduced/ Absent breathe sounds indicate pleural effusion, pneumothorax or collapse.				
• Whispering petriloquy 'Whisper 99' (increased in consolidation)				

Closing	Mark (0-4)			
• Thanks patient • Maintains patient dignity				

OSCES

Presentation	Mark (0-4)			
• Summarise their findings • Offers an appropriate differential diagnosis and management plan • Suggests appropriate inital investigations such as an ECG, CXR, PEF				

Follow On Questions

What would be your management of this patient?

ABCDE. Oxygen, sit up, nebulisers including salbutamol, steroids.
Early discussion with ITU for respiratory support is important. This case needs discussion with the surgical consultant in charge of her care and theatres as her operation will have to be cancelled.

What post-operative considerations are there specifically for this patient?

She is a heavy smoker, so there is an increased risk of respiratory complications (3-5x) including pneumonia, respiratory failure, atelectasis, ITU admission & sequelae.

How can you reduce these complications?

• Pre-operative optimisation- respiratory/anaesthetic review for elective cases, smoking cessation at least 4 weeks before surgery, chest physiotherapy pre and post-operatively
• Post-operative- adequate pain relief, sit upright, early mobilisation, chest physiotherapy, close observation in HDU/ITU is useful

Examiner's Overall Assessment		
Pass	Fail	Borderline

TOP TIPS

Be calm and systematic in your ABCDE examination, but use the examiner to direct you if they only require more detailed respiratory exam.

2.14 Shoulder Examination

Common Scenarios

Shoulder pain has multiple causes; common causes seen in the exam may include:

- Acromioclavicular joint sprain/arthritis
- Rotator cuff tear
- Subacromial impingement
- Instability/laxity (post-traumatic or congenital)
- Glenohumeral joint arthritis (in older patients)

 Candidate Briefing

Mr/Mrs A has presented to your outpatients clinic complaining of pain in his right shoulder. He/she is a normally fit and well builder in his 50s and tells you that he has a niggling pain on and off for many years but lately it has been constant and the arm feels weak. Please examine him as you see fit, present your findings to the examiner then answer his/her questions.

 Patient Briefing

You are a Mr/Mrs A, a 50 year old builder. You have a nagging ache in your arm, which has been present for some time but feels much worse recently, particularly when you reach above your head. When examined you should be minimally tender but have pain when raising your arm over your head, and some weakness/pain inhibition with resisted abduction.

Examiner's Mark Scheme

Introduction	Mark (0-4)			
• Wash/gel hands, explain procedure, obtain consent				
• Checks patient is comfortable and not in pain				

OSCES

Inspection	Mark (0-4)			
• From front, back and side • **Skin**: Scars, bruising/skin changes, swelling • **Muscle**: Asymmetry, deformity (winging of the scapula, wasting of deltoid) • **Bone & Joint:** Position of both shoulders (dislocations) • Remember to check the axillae.				

Palpation	Mark (0-4)			
• Temperature changes, tenderness or crepitus. • Standing in front of the patient: Palpate sternoclavicular joint, clavicle, acromioclavicular joint, acromial process, head of humerus, coracoid process, spine of scapula. • Standing Behind the patient: Check interscapula area for pain, feel for rotator cuff defects • Palpate supraclavicular area for LNs.				

Movement	Mark (0-4)			
• Active (Patient moves) then Passive (Doctor moves) movements. Fell for crepitus during passive movements.				
• **Flexion (0-180°):** Raise your arms forwards, up over your head.				
• **Extension (0-60°):** straighten yours arms behind you as far as possible.				
• **Abduction (0-180°)**: Move your arms away from the side of your body until your hands are touching.				
• **Adduction (0-45°):** Cross your arms over the front of your body.				
• **External Rotation (0-90°):** With your arms bent and elbows tucked into your sides move your hands outwards.				

• **Internal Rotation (0-90°):** Bring your hands together again from the position above.				
• **Internal Rotation in adduction:** Reach up behind your back and touch your opposite scapula.				
• **External Rotation in abduction:** Put your hands behind your head.				

Special Tests	Mark (0-4)			
Serratus Anterior Function • Scapula Winging: Ask patient to put hands with arms outstretched against a wall and push against it. Observe the scapulae from behind.				
Subacromial Impingement Tests • Hawkin's Impingement Test: place the shoulder out at 90 degrees with the arm hanging down, press back on the arm, internal rotation will cause pain with impingement • Copeland/Jobe's Test: The arm is held out to the side and patient internally rotates the shoulder as if pouring out a drink. Passive abduction in internal rotation is painful.				
Glenohumeral Stability Tests • Apprehension Test: With the patient seated or supine, externally rotate the shoulder. The patient demonstrates apprehension that the shoulder will dislocate, and will often resist.				
Acromioclavicular Joint • The Scarf Test: The scarf test is performed with the elbow flexed to 90 degrees, placing the patient's hand on their opposite shoulder and pushing back.				

Closing	Mark (0-4)			
• Thanks patient • Maintains patient dignity				

OSCES

Presentation	Mark (0-4)			
• Summarise their findings • Offers an appropriate differential diagnosis and management plan • Offers to examine the joint above and below and request initial radiographs				

Follow On Questions

Given the story and your examination findings, what are your differential diagnoses?

Subacromial impingement and rotator cuff tear/tendinitis would be likely in this demographic. He may ACJ or GHJ arthritis, or bicipital tendinitis. A longstanding labral tear is a possibility. He may have referred pain from a neck problem, such as nerve root compression.

What investigations would you like to perform?

Xrays would be useful in the first instance. An MRI is best for soft tissue pathology, with an MR arthrogram looking for labral tears.

What are the muscles of the rotator cuff? Where do they attach to the humerus?

The supraspinatus attaches to the superior greater tubercle, the infraspinatus and teres minor attaching posteriorly adjacent to each other. The subscapularis attaches to the lesser tubercle.

Examiner's Overall Assessment		
Pass	Fail	Borderline

TOP TIPS

"SITS" is a mnemonic to remember the rotator cuff muscles – supraspinatus, infraspinatus, teres minor and subscapularis.

2.15 Excision of a Lesion

Common Scenarios
This will typically be an actor with an artificial skin lesion attached to them.

 Candidate Briefing

You are the SHO in a plastics minor operations list. You have been asked to remove a skin lesion from Mr B's arm. Please proceed with the above task using the equipment provided.

This is a practical station. You should become familiar with the instruments used in a minor operations set.

The main instruments needed for this are:

Scalpel, toothed forceps, scissors, bipolar diathermy, needle holder, marker pen, ruler and scissors.

 Patient Briefing

You are Mr/Mrs B, you have presented to have elective excision of a small skin lesion. You should be generally cooperative and do not disturb the candidate, other than to ask about wound healing and when you need your stiches out.

OSCES

Examiner's Mark Scheme

Introduction	Mark (0-4)			
• Wash/gel hands, explain procedure, obtain consent				
• Confirms lesion and plan. Checks allergies and patient info				
• Marks appropriate lesion identifying excsion margins				

Skin Preparation	Mark (0-4)			
• Cleans skin with appropriate chlorhexadine solution				

Anaesthetic	Mark (0-4)			
• Anaesthetise with local anaesthestic using field block				

Scalpel Selection	Mark (0-4)			
• Selects an appropriate blade for the size of lesion such as 10-blade				

Scalpel Handling	Mark (0-4)			
• Attaches scalpel balde safely and securely				

Excision of Lesion	Mark (0-4)			
• Resects the lesion with an appropriate margin.				
• Uses a 3:1 technique to ensure an ellipse that will close. The ellipse should be three times as long as it is wide.				

Closure	Mark (0-4)			
• Choose a non-absorbable suture such as a 3-0/ 4-0 prolene on a cutting needle				
• Safely closes wound				

Sharps Disposal	Mark (0-4)			
• Safely disposes sharps into provided sharps bin				

Specimens	Mark (0-4)			
• Places lesion into pathology pot and labels form appropriately				

Follow On Questions

What are the safe doses of local anaesthetic?

3mg/kg 1% lignocaine
7mg/kg 1% lignocaine with adrenaline
2mg/kg bupivacaine

If you had used a non-absorbable suture when would you advise the patient to remove the sutures?

5 days for facial sutures
7 days for upper limb
14 days for lower limb

Does this patient require antibiotics?

No it is a clean procedure and antibiotics are not indicated

Examiner's Overall Assessment		
Pass	Fail	Borderline

TOP TIPS

There is frequently a lot to do in a short space of time in these stations. In addition, you often need to talk to the patient throughout. Rather than fully consent and explain to the patient, ask them if they have had everything explained and consented beforehand – if they say yes, you have saved a lot of time. The foam does not handle like skin, so do not worry too much if your excision looks horrendous, but you do need to demonstrate safe instrument handling and suturing, so concentrate on doing these well, even if you are unlikely to finish the station.

2.16 Varicose Vein Examination

Common Scenarios
Varicose veins should be pretty obvious on initial inspection and, given that they are both common and a stable chronic condition, they are an obvious choice for the exam.

 Candidate Briefing

Mrs B is a 55 year old female who you are asked to see in vascular outpatients. She is complaining of unsightly veins on mainly on her right leg and skin colouration surrounding them. Examine her legs as you think appropriate and present your findings to the examiner.

 Actor Briefing

You are Mr/Mrs B, a 55 year-old with varicose veins. You should struggle a little with the candidate's instructions – they need to be very clear in explaining what they would like you to do, particularly for the Tourniquet/Trendelenburg tests.

Examiner's Mark Scheme

Introduction	Mark (0-4)			
The candidate should: • Wash/gel hands, explain procedure, obtain consent • Ask for a chaperone and treat the patient with dignity at all times				
• Checks whether patient is in pain				

Inspection	Mark (0-4)			
• Inspect the patient from the end of the bed, commenting on general health and appearance				

• Stand the patient up • Thorough inspection of right leg, comparing to left leg as necessary to look for features of venous disease such as presence of varicose veins in LSV and SSV distribution, venous eczema, haemosiderin deposits, venous ulcers (gaiter region), scars				

Palpation	Mark (0-4)			
• Palpate varicosities and comment on evidence of thrombophelbitis				
• Feels for a transmittable thrill by palpating below a fixed point on the dilated vein				

Special Tests	Mark (0-4)			
• Auscultate over the sapheno-femoral junction (SFJ) for a bruit, caused by regurgitant flow after the calf has been compressed				
Tourniquet Test • The tourniquet test determines the level of venous regurgitation. • Lift the leg as high as comfortable to empty the veins, place a tourniquet, or press your thumb (Trendelenburg test) over the sapheno-femoral junction (SFJ), which is 4cm inferior and lateral to pubic tubercle. • Ask the patient to stand while you maintain the pressue over the SFJ. Rapid filling of varicosities means that incompetence lies below the SFJ (conversely control at this point means that the SFJ is the (main) problem). • • Repeat the test moving down 3cm at a time until varicosities controlled.				
Doppler • Use a handheld Doppler to identify regurgitant flow at the SFJ and sapheno-popliteal junction (SPJ)				

OSCES

Closing	Mark (0-4)			
• Thanks patient • Maintains patient dignity				

Presentation	Mark (0-4)			
• Summarise their findings • Offers an appropriate differential diagnosis and management plan • Suggests appropriate inital investigations such as venous duplex				

Follow On Questions

What investigation would you book for this patient to confirm your clinical findings?

Venous duplex

What criteria must a patient meet to be offered surgery on the NHS?

Evidence of skin changes secondary to varicose veins, pain inhibiting activities of daily living, episodes of thrombophlebitis or bleeding

How can varicose veins be managed?

Conservative: lifestyle changes such as weight loss or compression hosiery
Surgical: sclerotherapy, ligation and stripping, endovenous ablation

Examiner's Overall Assessment		
Pass	Fail	Borderline

TOP TIPS

 Examine the patient stood up, and have them turn around to face away from your, so that you demonstrate to the examiner a very thorough inspection. You could also mention completing your examination with history and examination of the abdomen and pelvis if there was any suspicion of venous compression by a mass lesion.

OSCES

3 VIVAs

VIVAS

3.1 | Aneurysms

 Candidate Briefing

A patient is admitted for an elective abdominal aortic aneurysm (AAA) repair. Please answer the examiner's questions related to the pathogenesis of this disease.

👓 **Examiner's Questions and Mark Scheme**

Mark

Define the term aneurysm

The abnormal localised dilatation of a blood vessel more than x1.5   /1
its normal diameter. For the abdominal aorta, the normal diameter is 3cm.

What are the risk factors for developing a AAA?

The candidate may wish to classify the different risk factors, as below:
Congenital: Male sex (9:1 female), family history (4-6x higher risk   /3
if sibling affected), Marfan syndrome, Ehlers-Danlos syndrome, cystic medial necrosis
Acquired: Smoking, hypertension, hypercholesterolaemia, arteritis (infective/inflammatory).

What are the risks of an untreated AAA?

Rupture and death, thromboembolism and "trash foot", renal dys-   /2
function, other aneurysms e.g. popliteal

How may a patient with a AAA present?

Asymptomatic/incidental finding – candidate should mention he
role of screening   /3
Symptomatic - pain, renal dysfunction.
Rupture.

Mark

What guidelines exist to guide management of AAAs?

The UK national AAA screening programme (NAAAS) recommends
ultrasound screening dependent on aneurysm size and rate of
increase.

/2

Do you know the diameter at which most vascular centres offer AAA repair?

5.5cm in men and 5cm in women or a rapid increase e.g. >5cm in
6 months (4-5.4cm carries a 1% rupture risk, rising sharply after
this). Evidence shows an advantage for survival over this threshold.

/2

What surgical options are available for AAA repair?

Open, endovascular, (laparoscopic).

/2

What are the advantages of endovascular aneurysm repair (EVAR) over open repair?

• Smaller incisions- decreased post-operative pain and risk of surgical site infection (SSI), better mobility.
• No peritoneal entry/bowel handling- decreased risk of inadvertent damage to other structures, minimised post-operative ileus.
• Decreased systemic insult.
• Shorter post-operative stay.
• Typically no need for intensive care admission.

/4

What are the disadvantages?

• Long-term data.

VIVAS

Examiner's Overall Assessment		
Pass	Fail	Borderline

TOP TIPS

 In the UK AAA screening program, men are invited for an abdominal ultrasound when they turn 65 years-old. If no aneurysm is found, then this does not need to be repeated, as the lifetime risk of subsequent AAA is around 1 in 1000. If the aneurysm is 3 - 5.5cm, the patient will be invited back at regular intervals for monitoring. Over 5.5cm will be offered elective repair. The DVLA should be notified of patients with an aneurysm >6cm, and patients should stop driving if their aneurysm is >6.5cm *(>5.5cm in bus or lorry drivers)*.

3.2 Brachial Plexus

 Candidate Briefing

Please study the below image of the brachial plexus, then answer the examiner's questions

---

 Examiner's Questions and Mark Scheme

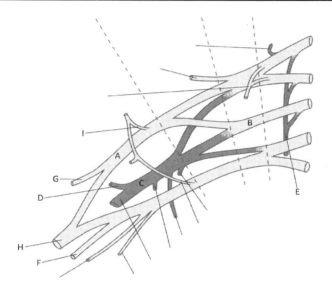

Mark

From which nerve roots is it formed?

/2

C5, 6, 7, 8, T1. Occasionally there are contributions from C4 or T2

Name structure G. What is its function?

This is the musculocutaneous nerve (C5,6,7), which supplies the muscles in the anterior compartment of the upper arm – biceps brachii, brachialis and coracobrachialis – as well as the brachioradialis in the forearm. It continues as the lateral cutaneous nerve of the forearm. These muscles flex the arm and supinate the forearm.

/3

VIVAS

Mark

Name structure H

/1

H is the median nerve (C5,6,8,T1).

Which muscles does structure H it supply in the hand?

It supplies the lateral two lumbricals and the muscles of the thenar /2
eminence – opponens pollicis, abductor pollicis brevis and flexor
pollicis brevis.

Which nerve is commonly injured in an anterior shoulder dislocation? Identify this on the image provided.

/2

The axillary nerve is at risk of injury due to its proximity to the hu-
meral head. It is labeled D on the image.

How might you test the sensory function of structure D?

Sensation can be tested over the 'regimental badge' area on the
lateral aspect of the shoulder. Motor function can be tested by ask- /2
ing the patient to abduct their shoulder using their deltoid muscle.

Name structure E. Which muscles does it supply? Describe what you will see with injury to this nerve.

/3

This is the long thoracic nerve of Bell. It supplies the serratus anterior muscle. Injury to this will cause winging of the scapula.

Demonstrate how you would test the radial, median and ulnar nerve function on the patient.

The radial nerve extends the fingers and supplies sole sensation
to the dorsal first webspace. The median abducts the thumb and /3
supplies sole sensation to the volar aspect of the index finger. The
ulnar nerve abducts and adducts the fingers and supplies sole
sensation to the medial aspect of the fifth finger.

Mark

Identify the ulnar nerve on the image. Through what region does it pass to enter the hand?

The ulnar nerve is labeled F on the image. It passes through /2
Guyon's canal to enter the hand.

What structures are A and C? Why are they named as such?

/3
A is the lateral and C is the posterior trunk. They are named for
their relationship to the axillary artery.

Examiner's Overall Assessment		
Pass	Fail	Borderline

TOP TIPS

Anatomy stations are difficult, because generally you either know
it or you don't. But a good tip, if you are struggling, is to ask the
examiner to move on and come back to the question later. They
may ask another question which gives away the answer, or jogs
your memory, but also it allows you to pick up all the other points,
rather than getting stuck on one question and missing out everything else.

VIVAS

3.3 | Burns

 Candidate Briefing

You are the surgical SHO on call and are called to ED to see a patient who has been involved in a fire at a local paintworks. He is phoned through by the ambulance crew as having large burns and in some distress. You await his arrival in ED with your registrar. Please consider your approach to this patient, then answer the examiner's questions.

Examiner's Questions and Mark Scheme

Mark

How would you manage this patient?

Candidate should describe the ATLS protocol for burns.
Assess airway- are airway burns a concern? Apply high flow oxygen & urgent anaesthetic review. Breathing. Circulation- 2x large bore cannula through unburnt skin, fluid resuscitation as per The Parkland formula*, catheterization. Disability- GCS assessment, analgesia.
NB: they should refer to stopping the burning process.   /2

The Parkland formula
Fluids for 24 hours = (4ml x kg x %burn)
50% of total in the first 8 hours
50% over the following 16 hours
This is a guidance only and further fluid resuscitation should be guided by urine output.

What threatens the airway in burns? What signs would you look for?

Thermal or chemical injury, as well as trauma if there has been an explosion/building collapse etc.   /2
Facial burns, singed eyebrows or eyelashes, soot around the mouth/nose, carbonaceous sputum and changes in voice. Stridor and respiratory distress are all worrying features of impending airway loss.

Mark

What would you do about these features?

A low threshold for anaesthetic involvement, early intubation and /2
ventilation. Supply high flow oxygen.

What aspects of burns injury can compromise breathing?

Thermal injury from smoke or hot air inhalation can cause direct /2
damage to the lungs. Burns to the skin of the chest may restrict
chest expansion, particularly if circumferential. These may require
emergency escharotomy.

What radiographic features in the lungs might you see?

May be normal or show evidence of pulmonary infiltrates. A pneu- /2
mothorax may be present in trauma.

If the chest film shows bilateral pulmonary infiltrates, in the context of a patient with high oxygen requirements, what would you suspect?

/4

ARDS: acute respiratory distress syndrome.

Where should this be managed?

/1

Intensive care for supportive treatment

What ventilatory strategies can be used to manage ARDS?

There is no clear consensus. High airway pressures may be /1
necessary. An inverse inspiration to expiration ratio is utilized, as is
prone ventilation.

Describe some general principles of burns dressing.

Burns should initially be dressed with a non-adherent dressing /2
what exactly depends what is to hand. Something like Jelonet is
ideal or even cling-film.

VIVAS

Mark

What cardiovascular problems can occur with severe burns and how are they managed?

The main issues relate to massive fluid losses from the burns. The candidate should describe a formula to guide fluid resuscitation i.e. Parkland.
Ask them to describe a formula if they don't volunteer one.
Parkland formula - see table above.

/2

What resuscitation fluid should you use?

Crystalloid such as 0.9% saline or Hartmann's.

/2

How can surface area of burns be calculated?

Should describe rule of 9s. Alternatively, 1 open palm and fingers surface area is approx. 1%.

/1

Describe the different grades of burn.

Erythema: eg sunburn – characterised by erythema and pain but no blistering. Not used in calculation of burn surface area.
Superficial partial thickness: erythema blanches on pressure, painful, blistering present.
Deep partial thickness: fixed red staining, can be painful or pain-less, blistering.
Full thickness: black/leathery/waxy insensate.

/4

Which burns warrant discussion with, or treatment in, a burns unit?

Greater than 15% of BSA in an adult and 10% in a child.
Any full-thickness burn or circumferential burns.
Burns to the hands, head, neck, perineum, feet.
Inhalation injury or any burn in the very young or elderly.
Associated trauma or co-morbidity.

/3

Examiner's Overall Assessment		
Pass	Fail	Borderline

VIVAS

3.4 | Cardiac Disease

 Candidate Briefing

You are discussing patients for the list tomorrow with one of the anaesthetists. One patient has some valvular heart disease and the consultant asks you some questions regarding this.

✍ Examiner's Questions and Mark Scheme

Mark

What is aortic stenosis (AS)?

Narrowing of the aortic valve, resulting in left ventricular (LV) hypertrophy & eventually failure. /2

Name some common causes of AS.

Causes include: Congenital e.g. bicuspid aortic valve (2%) or Acquired, e.g. degenerative calcification (majority), infection e.g. rheumatic fever, metabolic disease e.g. diabetes, Paget's /3

Why may aortic stenosis be problematic for deliverance of general anaesthesia?

• AS causes left ventricular (LV) outflow obstruction and a fixed low-output state with a secondarily stiff left ventricle. The LV does not compensate for a fall in systemic vascular resistance that occurs from use of general anaesthetic agents, so cardiac output does not increase and a downward spiral of severe hypotension, myocardial ischaemia & reduced contractility result.
• In addition, coronary perfusion is reduced at baseline due to the low-output state and minor changes in heart rate or cardiac output can have a clinically significant effect on myocardial ischaemia.
• Also the atrial contribution to cardiac output is proportionally much larger, up to 40% (normal is 20%).
• Arrythmias that may occur during anaesthesia may produce a critical reduction in cardiac output.

VIVAS

Mark

What steps are necessary for assessment of fitness of a patient with symptomatic aortic stenosis undergoing elective non-cardiac surgery?

• Anaesthetic, with or without cardiology assessment, including echocardiography and an ECG.
• Symptomatic patients are at high risk of sudden post-operative death so elective non-cardiac surgery should be delayed for valve replacement. The same applies for major elective surgery associated with large fluid shifts, e.g. thoracic, abdominal, or major orthopaedic.
• Asymptomatic patients undergoing minor/moderate surgery are generally safe when operated upon with careful monitoring and a low threshold for ITU/HDU admission.
• Correct any other cardiac disease such as atrial fibrillation pre-operatively. Prophylactic antibiotics sould be delivered at induction to reduce the risk of endocarditis.

/4

Which patients are at increased risk of infective endo-carditis from surgical procedures?

• Acquired valvular lesions
• Structural heart defects
• Prosthetic valves
• Previous history
• Hypertrophic cardiomyopathy

/2

Do you know of any guidelines for use of prophylactic antibiotics against infective endocarditis?

NICE 2008 guidelines. They recommend using antibiotics in procedures other than: dental procedures, genitourinary surgery or procedures confined to lower or upper GI tract, such as colonoscopy.

/2

Which are the most common bacteria associated with infective endocarditis?

• Staphylococcus Aureus
• Streptococcus Viridans
• Coagulase negative Staphylococcus

/2

Mark

For patients with prosthetic valves, what other peri-operative medication issues are there likely to be? How might you manage these?

• They are likely to be anticoagulated and will need this withheld and managed perioperatively. There are local & national guidelines for this.

/2

• For warfarin, stop 5 days before, cover with subcutaneous low molecular weight heparin when INR falls below range, then switch to intravenous heparin infusion during planned pre-op admission to hospital.

Examiner's Overall Assessment		
Pass	Fail	Borderline

TOP TIPS

 In such cases, where surgery may pose significantly higher risk to the patient than the usual, it would look good to say something along the lines of, *"having gathered all the information and con-sidered the risk, if operating was an option, I would put this to the patient, but ensure that I encouraged them to take an autonomous decision in possession of all the facts."* This shows that you are considering patient choice and autonomy as one of the fundamental principles of your practice.

VIVAS

3.5 | Colorectal Cancer

 Candidate Briefing

You are a surgical SHO in the colorectal clinic. Mr W is a 68-year-old who has been diagnosed with colorectal cancer. Please answer the examiner's questions on this disease.

👓 Examiner's Questions and Mark Scheme

Mark

What is the definition of an intestinal polyp?

A protuberant neoplasm of the intestinal lumen most commonly affecting the rectum & colon.

/2

Give two examples of different types of colonic polyp.

Benign: tubular adenoma, villous adenoma, Peutz-Jeghers polyps.
Malignant: polypoid adenocarcinoma, carcinoid polyp.

/2

Which of these have a higher malignant potential?

Adenomas- villous>tubular, size >1cm.

/2

What are the risk factors for colorectal cancer?

• **Congenital factors**: family history, inherited conditions- familial adenomatous polyposis (FAP), hereditary non-polyposis colorectal carcinoma (HNPCC), ulceratvive colitis (1% risk of malignant trans-formation per year), previous colorectal cancer.
• **Social factors**: smoking, diet- low fibre, high fat, high protein i.e. western. Age (uncommon <50).

/4

VIVAS

Mark

Define staging and grading of cancer

Staging: The process of determining extent of spread of a cancer. The stage generally takes into account tumour size, invasion through tissue of origin and confining wall, lymph node involvement and distant spread.

/2

Grading: A measure of cell anaplasia (reversion of differentiation) in the sampled tumor and is based on the resemblance of the tumor to the tissue of origin.

Name a staging system for colorectal cancer & describe its parts.

/2

Dukes (see below) and TNM

Stage	Features	5 year survival
A	Tumour confined to mucosa	90-95%
B1	Invades into muscularis propria	75-80%
B2	Through muscularis propria & serosa	60%
C1	Spread to 1-4 regional lymph nodes	45-50%
C2	Spread to more than 4 regional lymph nodes	
D	Distant metastasis	6-7%

Describe how colorectal adenocarcinoma spreads.

Lymphatic: run with the blood supply & drain into para-aortic nodes then to thoracic duct. Advanced cancer involves supraclavicular nodes.

Haematogenous: portal vein to the liver (30% have liver metastases on presentation). Other sites are bone, kidney, adrenals, lung.

/2

Transcoelomic: seeding throughout the peritoneal cavity, in 10% after resection

Direct: Colorectal cancers may invade directly into adjacent structures, such as the bladder, vagina and pelvic sidewall.

VIVAS

Mark

Explain the principles of management of colorectal cancer.

Discusses 4 of below (must discuss MDT & surgery):
• MDT including- surgeon, radiologist, pathologist, stoma care nurse, palliative care, OT, physio.
Once staging & grading done, discussion & planning of surgical resection/radiation/chemo/palliation
• Stoma site planning by stoma nurses
• Surgery- Curative surgery depends on stage & site. The aim is for clear resection margins (5cm proximal, 2cm distal, although opinion differs).
Rectal cancer (38% cases)- Total mesorectal excision (TME) offers best chance of cure. Upper rectum= anterior resection, lower rectum/anus= abdomino-perineal resection (APR).
• Anaesthetic assessment pre-operatively.
• Palliation: palliative surgery for tumour resection/debulking, bypass, de-functioning colostomy/ileostomy, stenting, radiotherapy especially of bone for symptoms relief.
• Chemotherapy- improves Dukes C survival, not for Dukes A, controversial in B.
• Radiotherapy- neither pre/post-operative have an effect on survival but reduce local recurrence, used pre-operatively to downstage tumours and increase chance of curative resection but makes planes more difficult to dissect.

/2

Examiner's Overall Assessment		
Pass	Fail	Borderline

VIVAS

TOP TIPS

Staging, grading, mode of spread *(blood, lymphatic, direct +/- transcoelomic)* and management *(MDT, surgery, chemo/radiotherapy, palliation)* are all much the same for any type of cancer. Know the definitions well and you can apply them to any cancer question.

3.6 | Endocarditis

 Candidate Briefing

You are the SHO on a cardiothoracic firm. A 69 year-old patient has been referred to your team by the cardiologists. She presented several months ago with shortness of breath and fever. Examination revealed a pyrexia of 38.5 and a systolic murmur. The patient reports no previous trouble with her heart. She was treated with antibiotics initially successfully, but has since progressed to left heart failure. The cardiologists have referred her for consideration of surgery. Please think about what might be going on, then answer the examiner's questions.

 Examiner's Questions and Mark Scheme

Mark

What do you think may be the cause of this patient's problems?

This combination of symptoms and signs is suggestive of infective endocarditis. Differentials include other causes of sepsis, such as chest or urine, and/or valvular heart failure.

/2

What is infective endocarditis?

Infective endocarditis is an inflammation of the endocardium of the heart, particularly the valves. Endocarditis may also be non-infective or marantic.

/3

Describe some common signs (not symptoms) associated with infective endocarditis

Fever occurs in 97%. A new or changing murmur is less common but helpful in making the diagnosis. Other signs include evidence of vasculitis, such as Roth's spots on the retinae, Janeway lesions (non-painful erythematous spots on the palms, caused by septic emboli), Osler's nodes (painful red raised lesions on the fingers, caused by immune complex deposition), stigmata of anaemia, splinter haemorrhages in the nails, other septic embolic phenomena, such as cerebral or epidural abscesses, splenomegaly and haematuria (due to glomeruolonephritis).

/4

VIVAS

Mark

What are the most common organisms involved?

Overall the most common organisms are Staph Aureus, Step Viridans and coagulase-negative Staph. Others include Pseudo- /4
monas spp., Clostridium septicum, Chlamydia psittaci and Candida albicans.

What comorbidities or preconditions may predispose to infective endocarditis?

Any comorbidity causing immunosuppression increases the risk of endocarditis, such as HIV/AIDS, Diabetes mellitus or alcohol abuse. Previous damage to heart valves is the greatest risk factor /2
– this may be as a result of previous rheumatic fever or degen- erative valvular disease. Other risk factors include artificial heart valves, intracardiac devices such as pacemakers, congenital heart defects, and extra-cardiac, such as haemodialysis or intravenous drug abuse.

What steps should be taken to investigate suspected endocarditis?

It is important to try and get a positive culture of the organism to enable directed treatment. This may be difficult to obtain from blood cultures, so at least three sets of cultures should be taken /2
from different sites before initiating empirical antibiotic treatment. Echocardiography can establish the diagnosis, with transoesopha- geal being more accurate than transthoracic. The classic findings are vegetations or intracardiac abscesses, as well as new regurgi- tant jets or abnormal valvular movement.

What surgery are the cardiologists referring for?

It is likely that this patient has developed valvular heart disease as a result of her endocarditis. Surgery would likely involve debride- /2
ment of infected material and valve repair or replacement, as appropriate.

What are the recommendations for antibiotic endocardi- tis prophylaxis before interventional procedures?

NICE no longer recommends any antibiotic prophylaxis prior to

Mark

upper or lower GI, genitourinary, respiratory tract or dental procedures. This is due to a lack of evidence for its use, and possible
risks of bacterial resistance.

/2

Which valves are most likely to be involved?

Left-sided endocarditis is most common regardless of the cause.
Rheumatic fever most often damages the mitral valve, so this is
most commonly affected. IV drug abusers are at increased risk of
right-sided endocarditis (usually the tricuspid).

/2

What would be the surgical approach to this area of the body? Describe it.

This would be most likely through a midline sternotomy, though
anterior thoracotomy or hemisternotomy is a possibility. Sternotomy
starts with a vertical skin incision over the middle of the sternum,
from the suprasternal notch to the xiphisternum. Dissection is
continued with diathermy through the superficial fat to reach the
sternum, which is scored with the diathermy. Blunt dissection is
used to create space at the supra sternal and to one side of the
xiphisternum, and sweep the pericardium back off the sternum as
much as possible. An electric sternal saw (or alternatively a Leb-
schke knife) is used to divide the sternum in the midline, exposing
the pericardium, which can then be opened to accesss the heart.

/4

Examiner's Overall Assessment		
Pass	Fail	Borderline

VIVAS

TOP TIPS

 NICE guidelines recommend against antibiotic prophylaxis for
endocarditis for most procedures, but for many operations this is
a moot point, as prophylactic antibiotics will be given anyway to
reduce the risk of other surgical-related infections. Endocarditis is
more common in those with previous valvular damage, so explore
these possibilities carefully when taking a history from a patient
with suspected endocarditis.

3.7 | Chest Trauma

 Candidate Briefing

You are the SHO on call and are called to attend the emergency department as part of the trauma team. A 26 year old gentleman has come off his motorbike at 80 km/hr and hit a tree. Your registrar and consultant are scrubbed in theatre for a laparotomy and have asked you to attend and assist as needed.

👓 Examiner's Questions and Mark Scheme

Mark

How would you initially assess the patient?

Approach the patient in an ccABCD manner as per ATLS protocol.

Control of major haemorrhage

C-spine control

Airway

Breathing   /2

Circulation

Disability

Secondary survey once primary survey is complete

Often as part of a trauma team you will be assigned a specific role within this assessment

The patient is maintaining their own airway but on assessment of breathing the patient has saturations of 90% on room air and he is complaining of pain in his chest. Describe how you would assess this patient.

Breathing should be assessed by looking at the respiratory rate,   /2
depth of breathing and the chest wall movements. The chest wall
should be assessed for any injuries or scars. The chest should be
percussed (as best able in a noisy trauma call!) and finally aus-
cultated. Supplements to the primary survey include a chest X-ray
and FAST scanning of the chest.

Mark

You suspect the patient has a pneumothorax on the right hand side. What clinical signs would you find?

Lack of movement of the right side of the chest
Decreased air entry on auscultation
Hyper resonance on percussion   /2
Possible tracheal deviation to the left
Decreased saturations
Low blood pressure and tachycardia
Possible bruising or evidence of injury to the right chest wall

Clinically the patient has a pneumothorax on the right hand side. What is your management?

The patient needs decompression of the pneumothorax. This is   /2
best achieved by finger thoracostomy, followed by insertion of a
drain

What kit is needed to insert a chest drain?

Chest drain (24Ch or above)
Underwater seal
Silk stitch   /4
Scalpel, Roberts/Artery forceps
Local anaesthetic such a 1% lignocaine (3mg/kg)
Green needle and 10ml syringe
Gauze and an occlusive dressing

What is the triangle of safety?

The area where it is safe to insert the chest drain. It is bordered by
the anterior border of the latissimus dorsi, the lateral border of the
pectoralis major and a horizontal line superior to the level of the
nipple.

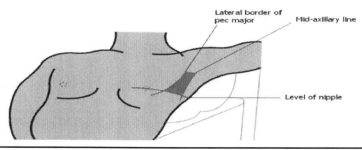

Lateral border of pec major   Mid-axillary line

Level of nipple

VIVAS

Mark

How would you perform a chest drain?

Verbal consent from the patient if possible
Ideally the patient should be sitting up at 45°C with their arm above their head
The drain should ideally be inserted in the 5th intercostal space just anterior to the mid axillary line
The area should be prepped with chlorhexidine and draped
Local anaesthetic should be infiltrated into the skin and along the tract of the drain into the pleural cavity if time permits
A 5cm incision should be made just above the 5th rib
Blunt dissection with the Roberts or Artery forceps through fat, fascia, outer intercostal muscle, inner intercostal muscle and innermost intercostal muscle to enter the pleural cavity   /4
A rush of air may be felt/heard once the cavity is entered
A finger should be inserted into the tract and a sweep performed to push the lung tissue away and any adhesions broken down
The drain should then be inserted into the chest along the tract
The drain should then be connected to the underwater seal
It should be secured in place with the silk suture
A purse string suture could also be placed in the wound to aid closure once the drain can be removed
An occlusive dressing should then be placed over the drain site.

The drain is inserted what you do next?

Order a CXR to assess the drain is in the correct position   /3
Leave on free drainage connected to the underwater seal until pneumothorax has resolved

Examiner's Overall Assessment		
Pass	Fail	Borderline

TOP TIPS

 Trauma is optimally managed as a team, with each team member designated a specific role, and one team leader standing away from the patient and having no active role other than to direct people. It is important to acknowledge this, as frequently everyone dives in and chaos ensues.

3.8 | Fistulae and Intestinal Failure

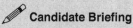 **Candidate Briefing**

A patient on your surgical ward has developed an enterocutaneous fistula following an emergency colorectal operation. On the ward round, your consultant asks you a few questions about this patient. Please answer the examiners questions.

Ꮖ Examiner's Questions and Mark Scheme

Mark

What is a fistula?

This is an abnormal communication between two epithelialised surfaces   /1

How is this different from a sinus?

A sinus is defined as a blind-ending tract communicating with an epithelialised surface   /1

What are the common causes?

Fistulae may occur for a multitude of reasons in many locations, but common aetiological factors include inflammation, relating to trauma, surgery, local sepsis/abscess, and malignancy.   /4

What are the results or sequelae of acute inflammation?

Acute inflammation may resolve completely, with no damage to the involved tissue. Alternatively it may proceed to suppuration, with pus formation; fibrosis and scar tissue formation; or chronic inflammation.   /2

VIVAS

Mark

What are the phases of acute inflammation?

These may be divided into Vascular, Cellular and Resolution or
Chronicity.
• Vascular phase: there is hyperaemia and increased vascular per-
meability, leading to influx of inflammatory mediators and immune
cells. This causes the erythema, swelling and pain of inflammation.   /2
In the succeeding
• Cellular phase: neutrophils and monocytes migrate to the site of
injury to phagocytose microorganisms and damaged tissue.
• Resolution
• Chronicity

How might an enterocutaneous fistula be managed?

SNAPP is a useful acronym:
• **Sepsis:** must be controlled, usually by drainage, either surgically
or radiologically. Antibiotics are an adjunct.
• **Nutrition**: fluid and electrolyte losses can be severe and should
be aggressively corrected. Parenteral nutrition is usually necessary
to ensure macro- and micronutrient requirements are met.
• **Anatomy**: particularly for complex disease eg Crohns, this pro-   /2
vides a roadmap for planning surgery, including distal obstruction
or strictures, additional abscesses or residual disease.
• **Protection**: of the skin – enterocutaneous fistulae will leak corro-
sive contents onto the skin and so stoma bags or similar should be
used to collect contents. Proximal diversionary surgery may also
be necessary.
• **Planned surgery**: restorative surgery should be delayed for at
least 3 months to allow abdominal adhesions to soften.

What factors may increase the chances of a fistula clos-
ing spontaneously?

Simple fistulas (not associated with malignancy or inflammatory   /2
bowel disease), with a low output (usually less than 200ml/day) in
patients with no or minimal comorbidities and good nutritional state
have the best chance of spontaneous resolution.

What amount of bowel is required to maintain normal
intestinal function?

/2

This depends a little on the presence or absence of colon. Less

Mark

than 100 cm of small bowel without colon or 50cm with colon will inevitably cause intestinal failure and reliance on parenteral nutrition.

What are some causes of intestinal failure?

These are multiple, and include:
• Massive resection for trauma or infarction   /2
• Fistulation
• Radiation enteritis
• Pseudo-obstruction or prolonged ileus

What are the risks of operating early on an intestinal fistula?

The risks may be classified as patient factors and surgical factors. The patient may be malnourished or under-resuscitated, which increases risks of any surgery. The underlying condition, such as Crohn's disease, may not be under control.   /4
In terms of surgical factors, allowing time for resolution of the inflammation in the peritoneal cavity is essential if possible. This allows acute adhesions to soften and make surgery possible. Before this time, the abdomen may be like "concrete" and make any operation difficult and dangerous.

What are the benefits of continuing some enteral feeding in a patient with intestinal failure requiring TPN?

Maintaining some enteral nutrition, either oral or by feeding tube,   /3
is beneficial in these patients. It has some psychological benefits in the first instance, but also helps contribute to maintenance of normal gut flora and normalisation of gastric pH.

VIVAS

Examiner's Overall Assessment		
Pass	Fail	Borderline

3.9 | Hypocalcaemia

 Candidate Briefing

You are the surgical SHO on call for general surgery and are called to review Mrs B who is recovering 6 hours after a partial thyroidectomy. She is complaining of paraesthesia around her mouth and in her hands and feet.

👓 Examiner's Questions and Mark Scheme

Mark

What are your initial concerns in someone with this brief history post thyroid surgery?

/2

Hypoparathyroidism leading to hypocalcaemia (most likely). Airway compromise secondary to haematoma, local anaesthetic toxicity.

What is the definition of hypocalcaemia?

/1

Adjusted serum calcium of less than 2.20 mmol/L

How is calcium stored in the blood?

In 3 states:
• bound to proteins (mainly albumin),
• bound to anions such as phosphate and citrate
• free unbound calcium. The free unbound calcium is the physiologically active component.

Mark

Name some signs and symptoms of hypocalcaemia

• Oral, perioral and acral tingling, 'pins and needles' sensation in hands and feet.
• ECG changes: prolonged QT, which can progress to torsade de pointes and ventricular tachycardia.
• Carpopedal spasm and tetany.
• Trousseau' sign- carpal spasm after inflating blood pressure cuff up to pressure greater than the patient's systolic.
• Chovsteks' sign- facial spasm illicited by tapping on the inferior border of the zygomatic arch
• Hyperactive tendon reflexes
• Laryngospasm
• Petechiae, initially present as intermittent spots but progress to purpura

/4

What are the common causes of hypocalcaemia?

• Hypoparathyroidism- either due to accidental surgical excision, damage to the glands at surgery or damage to the blood supply to the glands
• Vomiting
• Eating disorders
• Chronic renal failure
• Chelation therapy
• Vitamin D deficiency
• Osteoporosis treatment such as bisphosphonates or denosumab

/4

What vessel supplies the parathyroid glands?

Inferior thyroid artery.

/4

What does parathyroid hormone (PTH) do?

In response to low calcium levels, PTH induces the kidneys to reabsorb calcium.
The kidneys increase production of calcitriol (the active form of vitamin D).
This stimulates increased intestinal absorption of calcium and stimulates osteoblasts in bones to release calcium.

VIVAS

Mark

How do you treat symptomatic hypocalcaemia?

• 10% calcium gluconate IV over 10 minutes.
• Patient then needs regular calcium supplementation orally 1-2g/ day in divided doses.   /4
• Try to wean oral supplementation after 6 – 8 weeks.
• If needed for 6 months then likely to need lifelong calcium supplementation.

Examiner's Overall Assessment		
Pass	Fail	Borderline

TOP TIPS

 Consider other causes of this presentation, such a hyperventilation. You could make a comment to the examiner such as, *"I would first run through an ABC examination to exclude any immediately life-threatening pathology"* before moving on to discuss hypocalcaemia.

VIVAS

3.10 Open Fracture and Head Injury

 Candidate Briefing

You are the orthopaedics SHO on call and are asked to assess a 30 year old female who has fallen from a 5th floor window. The primary survey has been completed and you are about to start the secondary survey.

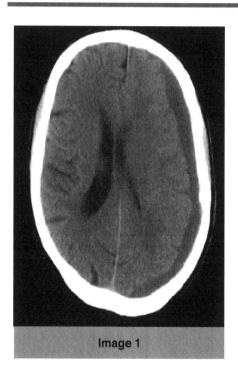

Image 1

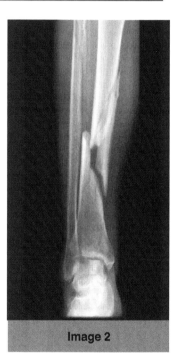

Image 2

VIVAS

✐ **Examiner's Questions and Mark Scheme**

Mark

What does the CT in image 1 show?

A subdural haematoma

/1

Mark

What is the management of a subdural haemorrhage?

The candidate should give an answer to include the following
points
ABCDE assessment   /2
Neurological observations
Correct coagulopathy
Discussion with on call neurosurgery service – may need transfer

The patient has sustained a head injury, what are the criteria for a head CT?

Definite indication:
Any new focal neurology
Seizure
Anticoagulation use such as clopidogrel, warfarin or rivaroxaban

High risk indications:
GCS less than 15 at 2 hours after injury
Vomiting (more than 2 episodes)
Open or depressed skull fracture   /2
Age 65 years or above
Basal skull fracture signs- haemotympanum, periorbital bruising/
racoons eyes, mastoid process ecchymosis/battle's sign, CSF
leakage from ear or nose

Moderate risk indications:
High risk mechanism of injury: Bull's eye on car windscreen, rolled
vehicle, ejection from vehicle, fall from a height of over 3 feet or 5
stairs
Pre trauma amnesia lasting more than 30 minutes

What is the management of a subdural haemorrhage?

The candidate should give an answer to include the following
points
ABCDE assessment   /2
Neurological observations
Correct coagulopathy
Discussion with on call neurosurgery service – may need transfer

Mark

What is the definition of raised intracranial pressure and possible management?

ICP >20mmHg in adults
Keep the head of the bed at 30° /2
Hyperventilation to aim for a pCO_2 30 – 35mmHg
3% hypertonic saline to keep a serum sodium of 155mmol/L
Mannitol can be used if serum osmolality >320 mOsm/kg
Surgical evacuation

During the secondary survey you notice an open wound over her right tibia and the patient is complaining of pain in this leg. What does the Xray (image 2) show?

/2

There is a comminuted fracture of the mid- and distal tibia, with segmental fractures of the proximal and distal fibula.

This is an open fracture. Do you know any grading systems for open fractures?

The commonly utilised system is the Gustillo Classification

Type1	wound <1cm
Type 2	wound 1cm – 10cm
Type 3A	>10cm wound, high energy, adequate tissue for coverage, segemental or extensively comminuted fractures
Type 3B	extensive periosteal stripping and requires free soft tissue transfer
Type 3C	vascular injury requiring vascular repair

/4

VIVAS

Mark

What is the management of an open fracture?

Based on guidance from BOA and BAPRAS
IV antibiotics as per local protocol, continue for 24hrs or until definitive soft tissue closure
Tetanus prophylaxis if indicated
Control bleeding   /4
Sterile saline soaked dressing
Splint the fracture for temporary stabilization
Discussion with a specialist centre with an orthoplastic service and early transfer
Debridement, fracture fixation and soft tissue coverage should occur simultaneously within 7 days

The patient goes to theatre in the morning for fracture fixation and soft tissue coverage as a joint case between orthopaedics and plastics. What are the reconstruction options available to ensure bone coverage?

/2

Employ the reconstructive ladder. The bone and metal work need to be fully covered so often the use of local tissue transfer is needed or a free flap.

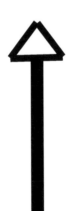

Free tissue transfer
Distant tissue transfer
Local tissue transfer
Skin graft
Direct tissue closure
Allow wound to heal by secondary intention

Examiner's Overall Assessment		
Pass	Fail	Borderline

3.11 | Ordering A Theatre List

 Candidate Briefing

You are assisting an elective general surgical list. Your consultant is running a little late and has asked you to order today's list and discuss with the theatre team. Below is today's list.

Please order the list and discuss with the examiner.

Name	Age	Procedure	Notes
Maurice Pike	70	Para-umbilical hernia repair	Latex allergy
Alan Jones	64	Left inguinal hernia repair	Pacemaker
Eileen Stewart	50	Laparoscopic cholecystectomy	MRSA
Carol Sharp	69	Excision of dermoid cyst from back	COPD, IHD, CCF
Sarah Pill	31	Laparoscopic cholecystectomy	Temp 38.5, diabetes

 Examiner's Questions and Mark Scheme

Mark

Candidates should go through each patient to highlight the specific details of each. The final order of the list is not as important as the explanation for it and understanding of impact of comorbidity on surgery.　/5

The candidate should acknowledge that they have limited information about the patients and need to investigate further.
The major operations should go first on a list where possible.　/5
They should mention updating the consultant.

VIVAS

Mark

Candidates should highlight the following issues:

Latex allergy

Ideally place first on the list and ensure staff aware to use latex free equipment or if not possible should go at the end of the list following a deep clean

/1

Pacemaker

Surgical and anaesthetic considerations. Should mention diathermy - avoid monopolar or minimal use with pad placed so the current pathway is as far away from the pacemaker as possible. Bipolar in short bursts distant from pacemaker. The pacemaker must have had a recent check - information includes pacing dependency, heart failure, any specific safety advice. Continuous ECG monitoring and discuss arterial line. There should be a crash trolley nearby for failure of pacing device.

/1

MRSA

If possible place last on the list and deep clean theatre following the case.

/1

COPD, IHD, CCF

Significant medical comorbidities here. Use of local anaesthetic if possible.

/1

Febrile patient

Intercurrent illness, cancel elective operation, go to explain and apologise to the patient, ensure medically well and will relist. Mention need to examine patient as may need discussion with and referral to an inpatient service depending on the underlying cause.

/1

Diabetes

Place early on list to minimize starvation. Refer to trust, diabetes society, ASGBI guidance. Elective minor surgery- take long-acting insulin/anti-diabetics in morning, then re-start when eating post-operatively. Can mention hypoglycaemia management. If the candidate does not mention the role of sliding scales, ask them about this.

/1

VIVAS

Mark

What is the difference between monopolar and bipolar diathermy?

Monopolar involves a current passing between the active electrode
on the tip of the instrument to an electrode plate on the patient.
The current is disseminated across a larger surface area than it   /2
originates in, so heat is not built up in the plate.
The bipolar current passes between the two tips of the instrument
therefore the heated area is much smaller & more defined. There is
no plate.

What are the complications of incorrect placement of the patient electrode and how can you minimize them?

The main complication is a burn to the patient, either by a surgeon
contacting the skin or incorrect electrode placement. You must   /2
place electrode on dry shaven skin away from bony prominences
and metal implants. Other risks include ignition of volatile gases &
liquids, arcing of a spark via other metal instruments resulting in
distant burns and pacemaker malfunction.

When reviewing a diabetic patient pre-operatively, what specific investigations would be useful to analyse their diabetic control?

                                                                          /2

Blood sugar measurements including diary, HbA1c, renal function.
Past medical history including renovascular, cerebrovascular, cardiovascular and peripheral vascular disease.

VIVAS

Examiner's Overall Assessment		
Pass	Fail	Borderline

3.12 | Pancreatits

 Candidate Briefing

You have recently admitted a 40 year old gentleman with acute abdominal pain radiating into his back. He is tender in the epigastrium, with voluntary guarding. His observations demonstrate a tachycardia of 110 bpm, but are otherwise normal. His initial blood results are shown below. Please answer the examiner's questions.

Hb	112	Ca	2.24
WCC	13.4	Na	136
Plt	368	K	4.7
Neut	11.9	U	8.1
		Cr	88
Amy	1140	Bil	34
CRP	125	ALP	250
		ALT	60
		Alb	34

 Examiner's Questions and Mark Scheme

Mark

What do you think is the most likely diagnosis?

/1

Acute pancreatitis

What is acute pancreatitis?

Acute pancreatitis is acute inflammation of the pancreas, characterised by abdominal pain and elevated pancreatitic enzyme levels in the blood and/or urine. Severe pancreatitis may involve necrosis of the pancreas.

/2

Mark

What test is typically used to make the diagnosis? Over what threshold is the diagnosis considered?

/4

Amylase is the characteristic marker. Over 3 times the upper limit of normal is considered diagnostic of acute pancreatitis.

What are some other causes of hyperamylasaemia?

Cholangitis, perforated peptic ulcer, mesenteric ischaemia, small bowel obstruction, acute cholecystitis, ectopic pregnancy and salpingitis

/4

What are the main causes of Pancreatitis? Name some other ones.

The most common causes are gallstones and excessive alcohol consumption. Other causes include trauma, steroids, mumps, auto-immune pancreatitis, scorpion venom, hyperlipidaemia, ERCP and drugs, such as thiazide diuretics.

/4

Do you know of any prognostic scoring systems for acute pancreatitis? Describe one.

The Glasgow score utilises 8 variables:
- PaO2 <8,
- Age >55
- WCC >15
- Calcium <2
- Urea >16
- LDH >600,
- Albumin <32
- Blood Glucose >10

/5

APACHE II scoring is relevant to patients on ITU. It utilises PaO2, temperature, MAP, pH, heart rate, respiratory rate, sodium, potassium, creatinine, haematocrit, WCC and GCS.
CT severity index scoring utilises the 5 point Balthazar grade of pancreatitis severity on CT and the 4 point Pancreatic Necrosis scale.
Ranson Criteria utilises an admission score based on Age >55, WCC >16, BM >10, AST >250 and LDH >350. At 48 hours scoring is completed, utilizing Ca <2, fall in HCT >10, PaO2 <8, BUN rise >1.8, Base Excess <-4 and fluid sequestration >6L.

VIVAS

Mark

How should this patient be investigated?

He should undergo relevant tests to complete his scoring – usually an ABG, LDH +/- AST levels and a BM. The first most useful investigation is an abdominal USS to see if gallstones are the cause. If LFTs are deranged but the USS does not confirm gallstones, an MRCP may be useful. CT is useful if other diagnoses must be ruled out, or if condition is worsening or CRP rising after 3 days.

/4

How should this patient be managed?

• The mainstays of immediate management are aggressive fluid resuscitation and analgesia.
• There is some debate over whether patients can be fed, but generally restricting them to clear fluids in the first instance is appropriate. It may be necessary to utilize other methods of feeding these patients, such as TPN or nasojejunal feeding.
• Antibiotics are not indicated unless there is evidence of pancreatic necrosis or extra-pancreatic infection.
• If gallstones are discovered to be the cause, ERCP may be considered early. The patient will require a laparoscopic cholecystectomy later down the line to remove the risk of recurrence.
• Alcohol cessation advice should be given if appropriate, and possible precipitating drugs should be discontinued.
• Acute surgery is rare, indicated for infected pancreatic necrosis. Necrosectomy is performed, sometimes with drainage or continuous post-operative lavage. These are high-risk procedures.

Examiner: if candidate does not mention antibiotics, ask them the role of these.

Describe some complications of acute pancreatitis?

These can be divided into local and systemic:
• Local include pseudocyst, phlegmon, necrosis, splenic artery pseudoaneurysm, splenic vein/portal vein/SMV thrombosis, haemorrhage, duodenal obstruction, CBD obstruction, progression to chronicity, ascites.
• Systemic include SIRS, ARDS, MOF, DIC, hypocalcaemia, hyperglycaemia, IDDM, pleural effusions, death.

Mark

What is the mortality of acute severe pancreatitis?

/1

This is in the region of 20%

Examiner's Overall Assessment		
Pass	Fail	Borderline

TOP TIPS

➕ *"PANCREAS"* is a useful mnemonic for remembering the components of the Glasgow score – PaO2, Age, Neutrophils *(white cells)*, Calcium, Renal function, Enzymes *(LDH, AST)*, Albumin, Sugar.

➕ Best practice guidelines for the management of acute pancreatitis are found on the British Society of Gastroenterologists website: http://www.bsg.org.uk/clinical-guidelines/pancreatic/uk-guidelines-for-the-management-of-acute-pancreatitis.html

VIVAS

3.13 | Post-Operative Chest Pain

 Candidate Briefing

Mr/Mrs S is a 62 year-old patient who underwent femoral-popliteal bypass for peripheral vascular disease of his/her left leg 3 days ago. The nursing staff have asked you to see him/her as they are complaining of chest pain. Observations are stable apart from a tachycardia of 120 beats per minute. An ECG shows this is atrial fibrillation. A chest x-ray is awaited. You have yet to see the patient, but the consultant wishes to ask you some questions about chest pain in the post-operative period. Please answer the examiner's questions.

 Examiner's Questions and Mark Scheme

Mark

What do you think may be going on here?

The candidate should give a reasonable list of differentials, bearing in mind the time elapsed since surgery. Differentials include angina/MI, atelectasis, LRTI, PE, aspiration pneumonitis, ARDS   /1

What investigations would you wish to perform?

Bloods – FBC, U+E, Cardiac enzymes, Calcium, Magnesium, Phosphate, ABG
CXR   /2
Serial ECGs
Possibly CTPA if suspicion reasonable for PE
Echocardiogram if suspicious for MI

What complications are typically associated with the immediate post-operative period?

    /3

Primary haemorrhage (eg inadequate haemostasis or slipped ligature), basal atelectasis, acute MI, shock/SIRS, oliguria/AKI

Mark

If the patient has had an MI, how should they be managed?

The management is a little more challenging given the patient's risk of bleeding and should be undertaken with discussion with both the vascular surgeon and the cardiologists.

Initially an "ABC" resuscitation approach should be undertaken. The patient can be given aspirin, GTN, oxygen and morphine reasonably safely, but other antiplatelets or anticoagulants carry greater risk of bleeding and should be discussed with a vascular surgeon.

/4

If the patient is having a STEMI, they may be appropriate for primary PCI, in which case this should be undertaken as soon as possible.

It may be sensible to involve an anaesthetist/critical care physician at this stage also.

How can their risk be reduced?

Tight control of blood pressure, cholesterol, sugars. Supervised exercise programs can be very useful. Patients may be considered for either CABG or Coronary Angioplasty/Stenting pre-operatively to reduce their risk.

/4

How can a patient's risk for surgery be assessed?

This should be undertaken in conjunction with the anaesthestists if major surgery is planned and/or the patient is potentially high risk. An adequate history should be taken, focusing on previous anaesthetics and past medical history.

Physical examination should assess the airway, along with the organ systems looking for evidence of systemic disease.

/4

Pre-op investigations include:
- ECG/exercise ECG
- Echocardiography/stress echo
- CXR if suspicion of chest abnormality
- Pulmonary Function Testing- spirometry.
- CPEX testing usefully combines cardiovascular and respiratory testing during exercise and is increasingly utilised.

VIVAS

Mark

What are some causes of pyrexia post-operatively?

• Lung complications occur early at POD 1-2, eg atelectasis, aspiration and pneumonia
• UTIs typically occur around days 3-5, often related to catheters
• DVTs and PEs typically appear at days 7 - 10
• Surgical site infections around days 5-7   /4

These are not set in stone and high index of suspicion must remain for any complication in a febrile post-operative patient. Some patients may develop pyrexia post-op that is due simply to the SIRS response from surgery, but other complications should be excluded first.

What are some risk factors for post-operative atelectasis?

Patient: obesity, smoker, immobility (elderly, disabled), elderly

/3

Surgery: thoracic/high abdominal incision, long operative time

General: poor pain management, prolonged bed rest/immobility, inadequate chest physio

Examiner's Overall Assessment		
Pass	Fail	Borderline

TOP TIPS

This is the sort of patient that should be escalated to seniors sooner rather than later. Vascular patients frequently have cardiac problems post-operatively, and present a challenge in terms of further management if anticoagulation is being considered. Most vascular surgeons would want to have this patient discussed with them prior to leaping into treatment – recognition of this fact and acknowledging it to the examiners shows insight and sensible decision-making.

3.14 | Post-Operative Oliguria

 Candidate Briefing

The details below are from a patient you have just reviewed, on the request of your consultant. Please discuss this case with them and answer their questions.

Mrs Kathy Salders
ID 11111
68 years old

Elective open repair of incisional hernia 2/7 ago
Extensive dissection with large wound, biological mesh, 1 drain
Incisional hernia in previous lower laparotomy wound 13 years ago

PMH-
Previous colonic cancer- T3N1M0, open resection, pre-operative radiotherapy, discharged from follow-up
HTN
DH- Ramipril 5mg, NKDA
SH- Lives with husband in house, secretary for surgical department

OE
BP 110/70, HR 90, RR 12, sats 99%a, afebrile
Alert in bed, orientated
Fluid chart- poor intake yesterday, better today, IVI stopped last night
Catheterised- falling UO last 6 hours, currently 15ml/hour
Drain- 75ml total serosanguinous

Dry tongue
Heart sounds clear, chest clear
Abdomen soft but tender across wound, dressing removed- clean wound, no palpable bladder
Catheter draining clear, concentrated urine
Calves soft non-tender

Bloods today- Hb 162, wcc 13, crp 30, urea 10, creat 120 (bl 100), k 4.0

Mark

Please give me a summary of your findings for this patient.

The candidate should give a succinct summary of the presenting /3
problem and identify the salient points, chiefly that the patient has
undergone a significant operation, has evidence of acute renal
failure on the bloods and is clinically dehydrated.

What is the current problem?

/1

Acute renal failure

Is there any treatment you will put into place immediately at the bedside?

• Management plan based on CCrISP principles
• Basic assessment of airway, breathing, circulation, disability and
exposure
• Ensure the patient has working and appropriate intravenous ac- /3
cess
• Ensure the catheter is not blocked, by flushing it with 50mls saline
with a bladder syringe
• A fluid assessment will guide replacement
• Hold any nephrotoxic medications

How can pre-renal and intrinsic renal failure distinguished on urinalysis?

/1

In pre-renal failure the function of the tubules remains, so urine has
a high osmolarity, high urea and creatinine and low sodium.

Would you consider diuretics?

A one-time challenge with a diuretic would be appropriate to see if
urine output can be increased following failure of increasing urine
output with an appropriate fluid challenge alone.

Mark

What are the potential complications of renal impairment?

• Hyperkalaemia leading to arrhythmia
• Pulmonary oedema
• Metabolic acidosis   /2
• Uraemia leading to encephalopathy
• Toxin build up of renally excreted substances e.g. of opioids
• Uraemic pericarditis
• Chronic renal impairment

The patient's renal failure does not improve initially and urinalysis reveals the presence of "muddy casts" in the urine. What process may be going on here?

/1

Muddy casts are pathognomic of acute tubular necrosis

What are the primary causes of acute tubular necrosis (ATN)?

These can be broadly divided into toxic and Ischaemic ATN:

/3

• Toxic is due to nephrotoxic substances, such as drugs like NSAIDs or Gentamicin.
• Ischaemic is secondary to hypoperfusion of the nephrons, such as during shock or renal artery stenosis.

What are the absolute indications for renal replacement therapy in acute renal failure?

There are four absolute indications:
• Hyperkalaemia   /3
• Pulmonary oedema
• Symptomatic uraemia
• Acidosis

VIVAS

Examiner's Overall Assessment		
Pass	Fail	Borderline

3.15 | Referral To A Trauma Centre

 Candidate Briefing

Miss S is a 24-year-old driver involved in an RTA overnight. She is currently on the general surgical ward in your local DGH following admission via A&E. Please read the notes below & then discuss with the consultant-on-call on the phone in the regional cardiothoracic centre.

Supplemental Material:
10 minutes to read this and make notes prior to viva.

1/1/15 23.00- ED consultant
Trauma call in resus. 24 yo RTA- car driver in head-on collision with lorry, both at 40mph. Cut out of car at 50 mins, GCS 15/15 at scene
On arrival-
A-   Clear
B-   RR 15, sats 94% 15l NRB, hyper-resonant PN on left side
20Ch ICCD placed- immediate release of air, underwater seal connected. Bruising to left thorax ant/posterior, multiple rib # suspected
C-   PR 100, BP 90/50, warm & pink, alert
HS normal
Bloods sent for FBC, U&E, LFT, CRP, clotting, G&S 4 units
Abdomen SNT
No pelvic injuries apparent
D-   BM 7, -ve BHCG urine, PERLA, GCS 15

Immediate treatment- 1L Hartmann's stat then 1h- BP rose to 110/60

CXR: Left pneumothorax with correctly sited ICCD, multiple L rib #

C spine cleared

Pelvic XR- No fracture

ABG (pre chest drain):
pH 7.36
PO2 9kPa
PaCo2 4kPa
Lactate 2
BE -2.5

ECG- NAD

Imp- 1. Traumatic pneumothorax 2. Responsive to initial fluid resus

PCA suggested for analgesia

2/1/15 00.45- ED consultant
Patient is clinically stable, sat up & talking.
Secondary survey clear. ABG improved.

Plan:
To the gen surgical ward for observation- accepted by gen surg SpR who reviewed pt in ED. PCA written up by anaesthetist.

02.30- Surgical F1
Bloods- Hb 110, egfr >90, clotting normal, all other bloods NAD
RV- Comfortable in bed. Has used PCA x4. Sats 98% OA, ICCD swinging & bubbling. BP 100/70, PR 95.

Plan- *Continue*

05.00- Gen surgical SHO
Called to the ward to RV patient as tachycardic 110.
Patient c/o some back/sternal discomfort, PCA not covering pain.
A-   Own
B-   Sats 97%a, RR 16, good expansion, R side clear, L decreased AE, bruising to thorax on left
C-   HR 110 regular, BP 90/40, cr 4s, warm peripherally, HS normal Abdomen SNT
D-   BM 7, PERLA, GCS 15
Plan- Stat IVI, I will DW SpR

RV by SpR- *For urgent CT thorax ?thoracic trauma*

06.00- *CT verbally reported by radiology SpR as widened mediastinum, left pneumothorax with drain in-situ, multiple rib fractures no other gross injuries, needs to discuss with consultant before full report but possible proximal descending aortic injury*

06.15 RV of patient- *BP has risen with 1L fluid to systolic 100 & maintained. HR 90. Still c/o chest pain.*
Plan- *NBM, needs DW cardiothoracics, patient & husband updated*

VIVAS

👓 Examiner's Questions and Mark Scheme

Mark

Introduction

The candidate checks who they are speaking to on the telephone, introduces themselves appropriately and states why they are calling.   /2

The candidate gives a succinct summary of the events and the reason for calling such as:

"We have a 24 year old female who presented to ED last night at 11pm following a head on collision with a lorry at 40mph. She was extricated from the car after 50 minutes and was GCS 15 at the scene. She was assessed in ED resus by the ED consultant and found to have a left sided pneumothorax for which a chest drain was inserted. A CXR confirmed the drain's correct position as well as multiple left sided rib fractures. A secondary survey has been performed and no other injuries have been found except for the chest trauma. Her c-spine has been cleared. She was then transferred to the general surgical ward with a PCA for analgesia. Everything was ok until 5am when she complained of increased sternal and back pain and had become tachycardic at 110bpm. She was seen by my registrar who was concerned about thoracic trauma. A CT aorta at 6am has been verbally reported as a left pneumothorax, rib fractures and a widened mediastinum which they are concerned represents a descending aortic injury. I am calling for advice and wonder whether I can arrange for transfer of the patient to your centre as we do have any cardiothoracic service here please."   /6

The cardiothoracic consultant then proceeds to question the candidate further, requesting if the patient is currently stable?

/1

Candidate: "The patient has received a further 1L fluid bolus and her BP has come up to 100 systolic and her heart rate has decreased to 90 bpm at last assessment."

CT Consultant: "How much fluid has the patient received in total?"

/2

Candidate: "They have received 2L in fluid boluses and then maintenance fluid with the PCA."

Mark

CT Consultant: "What did the patient's latest blood gas show?"

Candidate: "The only blood gas I have documented is one done initially in ED prior to the ICCD insertion. This showed the patient to be hypoxic with a PaO2 of 9kPa but a normal pH and a lactate of 2. I will do another once I finish this phone call."

/2

CT Consultant: "What type of chest drain does she have?"

Candidate: "She has a 20 french left sided chest drain with an underwater seal inserted with an open technique. Its position has been checked on a CXR."

/2

CT Consultant: "You said she was tachycardic and hypotensive what have the bloods shown? Is her Hb ok?"

Candidate: "It is documneted that her Hb at 2.30am was 110, we do not have a previous sample to compare. I will check them myself after this conversation to make sure this is correct."

/2

CT Consultant: "Are there any other injuries? What imaging has she had"

Candidate: "I haven't examined the patient myself but it is documented that there are no other injuries found on the primary or secondary survey except the chest trauma. She has had a CXR, c-spine XRs, a pelvic XR and a CT thorax."

/2

CT Consultant: "What did the CT scan show?"

Candidate: "It has been reported as a widened mediastinum, left pneumothorax with drain in-situ and multiple rib fractures. No other gross injuries. It needs to be discussed with the consultant before the full report is issued but there is a proximal descending aortic injury."

/2

VIVAS

Mark

CT Consultant: "Sounds like we need the patient here in case she needs surgery. Could you please transfer the images to us and make sure she has two labelled group and saves and a copy of her notes with her.

I am happy to accept her transfer if she is haemodynamically stable.

What did I ask you to do prior to her transfer?" /2

Candidate: "You asked me to transfer the images of our CT thorax to yourselves, send the patient with two labelled group and saves and a copy of her admission notes so far. Thank you for accepting the patient. I shall arrange her transfer now."

Examiner's Overall Assessment		
Pass	Fail	Borderline

TOP TIPS

A lot of this station is testing your ability to communicate clearly and concisely, and not get rattled under pressure. The person on the other end of the phone may try and be deliberately difficult – try to work around this and do not let it put you off. Stick to your guns, but equally do not make up information that you do not have. Simply apologise, admit matter-of-factly that you do not have that information but you will do your best to get it ASAP.

VIVAS

3.16 | Sepsis

 Candidate Briefing

You have just referred a patient to the intensivists with severe bilary sepsis. They are now on ITU and the ITU consultant asks you some questions about sepsis. Please enter the station and answer the consultant's questions.

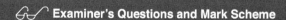

Examiner's Questions and Mark Scheme

Mark

What are the SIRS criteria? Define sepsis and septic shock.

• WCC <4 or >12
• RR >20
• HR >90
• Temp <36 or >38   /3
Two or more indicates the presence of SIRS.

Sepsis is SIRS plus a source of infection.
Septic shock is sepsis with hypotension unresponsive to IV fluids

What are the components of the 'Sepsis Six'?

• High flow oxygen
• Intravenous fluids
• Intravenous antibiotics   /1
• Catheterisation with urine output monitoring
• Blood cultures
• Lactate level

Define severe sepsis?

Sepsis with evidence of end organ dysfunction   /1

VIVAS

Mark

Name some causes of SIRS other than infectious

• Burns
• Pancreatitis
• Trauma   /3
• Anaphylaxis
• Haemorrhage
• Ischaemia
• Surgery

What is the role of procalcitonin in sepsis?

Procalcitonin levels rise particularly in response to infection of
bacterial origin;
a recent meta-analysis found reasonable evidence to support its   /2
use as a biomarker of bacterial sepsis, distinguishing this from
SIRS. Its sensitivity and specificity are around 76% and 70%,
respectively

Describe early goal-directed therapy?

EGDT is utilised in critical care and is the practice of invasively
monitoring and aggressively treating disturbances in cardiovascu-
lar status, particularly targeting cardiac preload, contractility and
afterload.
If there is poor response to initial fluid boluses, then targets are set:
• CVP of 8-12mmHg   /3
• SVC O2 saturation of >70% (or lactate normalisation)
• MAP > 65mmHg
• Urine output >0.5ml/kg/h.
Use of crystalloids, blood products to correct anaemia, inotropes
and vasopressors are key to achieving these goals. When correctly
performed, substantial reductions in mortality are seen.

What is Noradrenaline? How is it useful in septic shock?

Noradrenaline is an alpha-adrenergic catecholamine and works
as a vasopressor. It acts on alpha 1 and 2 receptors in vascular
smooth muscle, causing widespread vasoconstriction and increas-   /1
ing blood pressure.
It is therefore useful in vasodilatory states, such as sepsis and
anaphylaxis.

VIVAS

Mark

What is ARDS?

Acute respiratory distress syndrome is a syndrome defined by
type 1 respiratory failure and non-cardiogenic pulmonary oedema.
It results from widespread inflammation in the lungs, with cyto-
kine release, pulmonary capillary permeability and impairment of   /2
endothelial barriers, loss of surfactant, alveolar fluid accumulation
and fibrotic changes. It occurs within 1 week of initial insult and
characteristic CXR findings are bilateral pulmonary infiltrates no
explained by other pathology.

What is disseminated intravascular coagulation?

DIC is a consumptive coagulopathy resulting from widespread activation of the clotting system, leading to microvascular thrombosis,   /1
consumption of clotting factors and platelets and activation of the
fibrinolytic system. Coagulopathy and bleeding result. DIC occurs
as a result of underlying pathology, such as sepsis or burns.

What is the role of lactate measurement in Sepsis? Should this be arterial or venous?

Elevated lactate is an independent predictor of mortality and so   /3
can be used prognostication, as well as identifying patients in
whom higher levels of care may be warranted.

Examiner's Overall Assessment		
Pass	Fail	Borderline

VIVAS

TOP TIPS

 Sepsis is a very common topic, you should learn it in detail, using
the 'Surviving Sepsis' guidelines found at: http://www.survivingsep-
sis.org

3.17 | Skin Cancer

Candidate Briefing

You are the plastics SHO and are about to begin the morning minor ops list for skin cancer excision. Please answer the examiners questions about skin cancer management.

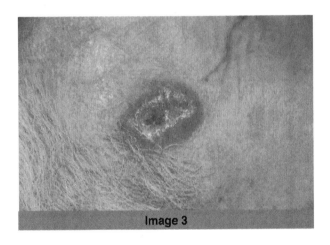

Image 3

Examiner's Questions and Mark Scheme

Mark

What are the main three types of skin cancer?

- Malignant melanoma
- Basal cell carcinoma
- Squamous cell carcinoma

/3

Mark

For each type, what cell type becomes malignant?

• Malignant melanoma: uncontrolled growth of pigment cells called melanocytes. Found in the basal layer of the epidermis.

• Squamous cell carcinoma: uncontrolled growth of keratinising cells of the epidermis. Locally invasive and has the potential to metastasise.

/3

• Basal cell carcinoma-locally invasive malignant epidermal tumour of the basal cells

What are the risk factors for developing a skin cancer?

• Ultraviolet radiation from sun exposure
• Fair skin, Fitz-Patrick skin types I and II
• Ionizing radiation and artificial UV radiation
• Smoking
• HPV infection increases the risk of squamous cell carcinoma
• Congenital melanocytic naevi greater than 20 mm in size
• Chronic non-healing wounds (Marjolin's ulcer) can develop into squamous cell carcinoma
• Immunosuppressive medications such as cyclosporine A and azathioprine

/4

The first case is a suspected melanoma. What margins of excision should you use?

Margins of excision should depend on Breslow thickness:

Breslow Thickness	Excision Margin
Melanoma in situ	5 mm
<1mm	1 cm
1.01 – 2mm	1 – 2 cm
2.1 – 4mm	2 – 3 cm
>4mm	3 cm

/5

VIVAS

Mark

What grading system do you use to advise on the prognosis of melanoma?

Clark's level and Breslow depth

Clark Level	Anatomical invasion	5-year survival rate
Level I	Intraepidermal dermal growth with intact basement membrane	>95%
Level II	Invasion of the papillary dermis	95%
Level III	Tumour involvement filling the papillary dermis and involvement of the junction between the papillary and reticular dermis	80 – 85%
Level IV	Invasion into the reticular dermis	80 – 85%
Level V	Invasion into the subcutaneous fat	55%

/4

What is lesion shown in image 3?

This is likely to be a Basal Cell Carcinoma

/1

Typical features of a basal cell carcinoma: rolled edge, pearly appearance and telangiectasia, typically seen on the face and hands)

What are the management options?

Surgical excision: With a 5mm margin will give a 95% clearance rate in tumours <20mm and 82% clearance in larger tumours

Non-surgical treatment with topical 5% imiquimod is suitable for small basal cell carcinomas being used for a 6 week course

/3

Radiotherapy is also an option for primary BCC tumours where the patient is unsuitable for surgery, there is recurrent disease or as an adjuvant therapy.

VIVAS

Mark

Describe how would you assess a skin lesion if it presented to clinic?

History:
Duration of the lesion
Change in size
Change in colour
Change in shape
Symptoms- itching, bleeding /4

Examination:
Site
Size (maximum diameter)
Elevation (flat, palpable, nodular)
Irregular margins or Irregular pigmentation
Ulceration present
Local lymph nodes present

Examiner's Overall Assessment		
Pass	Fail	Borderline

TOP TIPS

 Skin lesions can all look very similar to the untrained eye. Spend some time looking at as many different ones as possible, either in clinic or in textbooks/online along with the descriptions, so that you get a better feel for what actually constitutes a pearly appearance, rolled edge etc.

VIVAS

3.18 Stomas

 Candidate Briefing

You are on a surgical ward round and your consultant is reviewing a patient who is day 1 post-op emergency Hartmann's procedure.

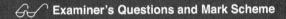 **Examiner's Questions and Mark Scheme**

Mark

What type of stoma would you expect to see post-Hartmann's procedure

/3

End colostomy

When is an emergency Hartmann's procedure used?

A Hartmann's is indicated for rectosigmoid pathology requiring resection when it is not possible to perform primary anastomosis because of concerns of anastomotic leak from:

/3

- Gross contamination
- The blood supply is doubtful
- Presence of infection or perforation

What is the definition of a stoma?

An opening either natural or surgically created, which connects a part of the body to the external environment

/5

What are the possible complications of stomas?

Acute: ileus, high output, retraction, stoma necrosis, bleeding, wound infection, leaking, skin irritation
Intermediate: stoma stenosis, prolapse, parastomal hernia, peristomal varices in patients with portal hypertension
Long-term: parastomal hernia, psychological concerns

/3

VIVAS

Mark

What are the differences between an ileostomy and a colostomy?

	Ileostomy	Colostomy
Site	Usually right iliac fossa	Usually left iliac fossa
Shape	Spouted. This is due to caustic nature of the effluent which irritates the surrounding skin and the spout aims to minimise this.	Flush with the skin
Effluent	Small bowel contents (liquid)	Semi-solid to solid faeces
Output	Low output: 500ml/day	
High output: 1 litre/day	200- 300ml/day	

/3

What other stomas do you know?

- Nephrostomy
- Jejunostomy
- Gastrostomy
- Cecostomy
- Urostomy (ileal conduit)
- Laparostomy

/4

When would you look to reverse an ileostomy?

Once the reason for the ileostomy creation in the first place has been treated, such as colonic cancer resection unsuitable for primary anastomosis so covering ileostomy used. Cancer treatment should have been concluded. Usually earliest at 3 months post creation. Similarly for creation of an ileo-anal pouch in Crohn's disease- a covering ileostomy is used for 8 – 10 weeks before reversal.

/4

VIVAS

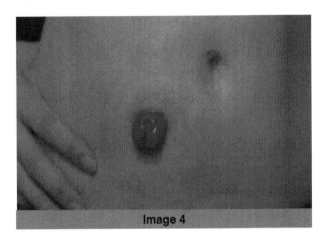

Image 4

Mark

Regarding figure 4. What type of stoma is this most likely to be?

/1

An ileostomy. As it is spouted and located in the right iliac fossa

Examiner's Overall Assessment		
Pass	Fail	Borderline

TOP TIPS

There are obvious multiple types of gastrointestinal stoma, but don't forget the definition of a stoma – *"a natural or artificial opening from a hollow viscus to the outside world"* – means that many other things can be considered stomas, including the mouth. Other artificial stomas include tracheostomies and cholecystostomies.

3.19 | Testicular Tumours

 Candidate Briefing

You are currently working on a Urology firm and have been helping the consultant in clinic. You have seen a 21 year-old man who underwent surgery for testicular cancer 2 months ago and has returned for follow-up. The consultant sees the patient himself then discusses the patient with you. Please enter the station and answer his questions

---

 Examiner's Questions and Mark Scheme

Mark

What surgery is he likely to have undergone?

Treatment for testicular cancer is a radical (inguinal) orchidectomy. Retroperitoneal lymph node dissection is sometimes performed, but is controversial.

/1

Briefly outline the approach to an inguinal orchidectomy.

This is very similar to that undertaken for an open inguinal hernia.
• An incision is made over the inguinal canal, using the ASIS and pubic tubercle as landmarks.
• Dissection is continued down to the external oblique, which is incised and then split in the line of its fibres.
• This reveals the cord in inguinal canal, which is dissected free, clamped and the testis delivered from the scrotum into the wound.

/2

How may testicular cancer present?

The most common presentation is with a painless lump in the testicle. Other features include haematospermia, testicular pain or a dragging sensation, hydrocele, gynaecomastia and other features of malignant spread.

/2

VIVAS

Mark

What different types of tumour are there?

• Seminomas   /2
• Non-Seminomatous Germ Cell Tumours (NSGCTs). This includes
teratomas and yolk sac tumours.

What risk factors exist for testicular cancer?

• Cryptorchidism/maldescended testis
• Family history
• Male infertility   /2
• Infantile hernia
• Testicular microlithiasis
• Klinefelter's syndrome

What is the lymphatic drainage of the scrotum and the testes? Why is this important in planning surgical procedures?

The scrotum drains to the inguinal lymph nodes, while the testes
drain to para-aortic lymph nodes in the retroperitoneum. This is
important for both primary surgery and also determining spread
of cancers. Biopsies should general not be taken percutaneously   /4
through the scrotum as they risk seeding into the scrotal
skin and thus giving two routes for metastatic lymphatic spread,
rather than one.
Similarly, radical orchidectomy should be undertaken through an
inguinal approach, to ensure complete excision of the testes with
attached spermatic cord, to minimize distant spread.

What age groups are typically affected by testicular cancer?

                                                                                               /1
It is most common in ages 20-39 and is almost never seen below
the age of 15.

What is its prognosis?

Prognosis is excellent, with a mean 5 year survival of 95%. With   /1
metastatic spread, this reduces to around 75-80%, with chemo-
therapy generally being very effective.

Mark

How would you investigate someone presenting in clinic with a testicular lump?

• Scrotal ultrasound is the most appropriate initial investigation.
• If cancer is suspected, a CT chest, abdomen and pelvis should be used to stage the disease.
• Tumour markers (B-HCG, AFP, Prolactin) should be taken prior to surgery and, if raised, after surgery. A persistently raised post-operative level suggests residual (metastatic) disease.
• Definitive diagnosis is via histology and for the reasons above should be via radical inguinal orchidectomy.
• Management is undertaken in a testicular cancer MDT.

/2

In a man presenting with a lump in his scrotum, what differentials should be considered?

• Epididymitis
• Epididymal cyst
• Hydrocoele
• Varicocoele
• Inguinoscrotal hernia
• Sebaceous cyst

/1

What is the role of medical/oncological treatments for testicular cancer?

Metastatic disease is treated with cisplatin-based chemotherapy.

Seminomas are radiosensitive and abdominal lymph nodes may be irradiated to treat occult metastases, if macroscopic disease is confined to the testis.

/3

Localised teratomas can be monitored with CT scans and tumour marker testing without adjuvant therapy.

Testicular lymphoma will be managed by the usual haemotological regimens.

VIVAS

Examiner's Overall Assessment		
Pass	Fail	Borderline

3.20 The Thyroid

 Candidate Briefing

You are working on an endocrine firm. Having seen a patient in clinic complaining of heat intolerance, weight loss and a neck lump, your consultant asks you some questions about the thyroid. Please answer the examiner's questions.

Examiner's Questions and Mark Scheme

Mark

Where is the thyroid gland found?

The thyroid gland is found in the anterior neck, deep to the pretracheal fascia, anterior to the thyroid and cricoid cartilages and the first few cartilaginous rings of the trachea.

/1

Describe its basic morphology and anatomy.

It consists of two lobes with a connecting isthmus, from which may arise a third 'pyramidal' lobe. Each lobe is about 5 x 3 x 2 cm. It is attached firmly to the underlying cartilages of the larynx and trachea. The infrahyoid muscles cover it anteriorly and the sternocleidomastoids cover it laterally. Microscopically it consists of follicles, surrounded by follicular cells, with parafollicular cells scattered around these.

/3

What is its blood supply? Where do these vessels arise?

The blood supply is by the superior thyroid artery, a branch of the external carotid, and by the inferior thyroid artery from the thyrocervical trunk, itself a branch of the subclavian. There may also be a thyroid ima artery supplying the isthmus, arising from the brachiocephalic trunk.

/2

VIVAS

Mark

Describe the venous drainage of the thyroid.

Venous drainage is via the superior and inferior thyroid veins. /2
The superior drain into the internal jugular; the inferior into the left
brachiocephalic vein.

What is the function of the thyroid gland?

The thyroid follicles produce the hormones Thyroxine (T4) and Tri-
iodothyroinine (T3), which play several important roles in metabolism and development.
During development maturation of the brain is crucially reliant on /3
T3. In life, T3 and T4 are vital for increasing metabolism, for growth
and development and also during times of stress.
The parafollicular cells produce the hormone Calcitonin, which
serves to lower the level of serum calcium.

Describe the physiology of the production of thyroxine and tri-iodothyronine.

T4 and T3 are formed from iodinated Tyrosine. Tyrosine is found
free and also as part of Thyroglobulin in the follicles in the thyroid.
The enzyme Thyroid Peroxidase (TPO) serves to bind iodine to /3
Tyrosine. Upon stimulation by Thyroid-Stimulating Hormone (TSH),
the follicular cells resorb Thyroglobulin from the follicles and cleave
the iodinated Tyrosine residues from it, to form T3 and T4 (so-
called because T3 has 3 iodide ions bound to it, where as T4 has
4).

Describe the feedback pathways involved in thyroid hormone release.

Higher control is at the level of the cerebrum. Increased require-
ment for thyroid hormone production (such as cold exposure) is
detected by the hypothalamus, which releases Thyrotropin-Releas- /3
ing Hormone (TRH). This acts on the anterior pituitary, stimulating
TSH production. TSH then acts on the thyroid. High levels of T4
suppress TSH and TRH production, in a negative feedback loop.

VIVAS

Mark

What dietary trace element is necessary for adequate thyroid function?

/1

Iodine is essential; deficiency leads to hypothyroidism.

Describe the symptoms and signs of hyperthyroidism.

Hyperthyroidism is characterised by excessive sympathetic activity. Patients will complain of anxiety, irritability, heat intolerance, fatigue, weight loss, palpitations, sweating, increased appetite, diarrhoea or a neck mass. Signs depend a little on the cause, but may include tachycardia, hypertension, arrhythmias, tremor, thin skin, dry hair, delirium, eye signs such as proptosis or exophthalmos, and a goitre.

/2

What is the most common cause of hyperthyroidism? Name another.

Graves' disease.
Other causes include toxic multinodular goitre or thyroid adenoma, thyroiditis or iatrogenic, for example excessive levothyroxine consumption or amiodarone use.

/2

Examiner's Overall Assessment		
Pass	Fail	Borderline

TOP TIPS

 Don't forget the Parafollicular cells within the thyroid that produce Calcitonin. It is important to distinguish these from the Parathyroid glands, situated in the posterior aspects of the thyroid lobes but histologically distinct from the thyroid itself. These produce Parathyroid Hormone, which is more important in calcium metabolism in the human.

VIVAS

Printed in Great Britain
by Amazon